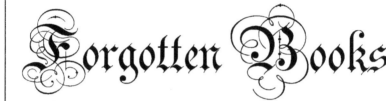

ISBN 978-1-332-03177-1
PIBN 10272365

# 1 MONTH OF
# FREE
# READING

## at

## www.ForgottenBooks.com

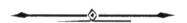

By purchasing this book you are eligible for one month membership to ForgottenBooks.com, giving you unlimited access to our entire collection of over 1,000,000 titles via our web site and mobile apps.

To claim your free month visit:

www.forgottenbooks.com/free272365

English
Français
Deutsche
Italiano
Español
Português

# www.forgottenbooks.com

**Mythology** Photography **Fiction**
Fishing Christianity **Art** Cooking
Essays Buddhism Freemasonry
Medicine **Biology** Music **Ancient**
**Egypt** Evolution Carpentry Physics
Dance Geology **Mathematics** Fitness
Shakespeare **Folklore** Yoga Marketing
**Confidence** Immortality Biographies
Poetry **Psychology** Witchcraft
Electronics Chemistry History **Law**
Accounting **Philosophy** Anthropology
Alchemy Drama Quantum Mechanics
Atheism Sexual Health **Ancient History**
**Entrepreneurship** Languages Sport
Paleontology Needlework Islam
**Metaphysics** Investment Archaeology
Parenting Statistics Criminology
**Motivational**

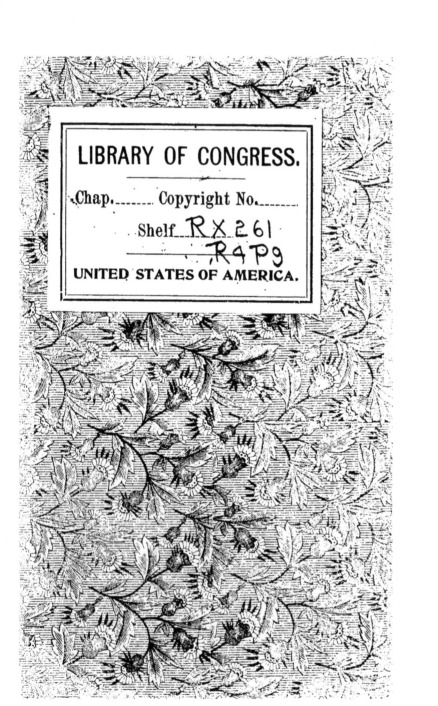

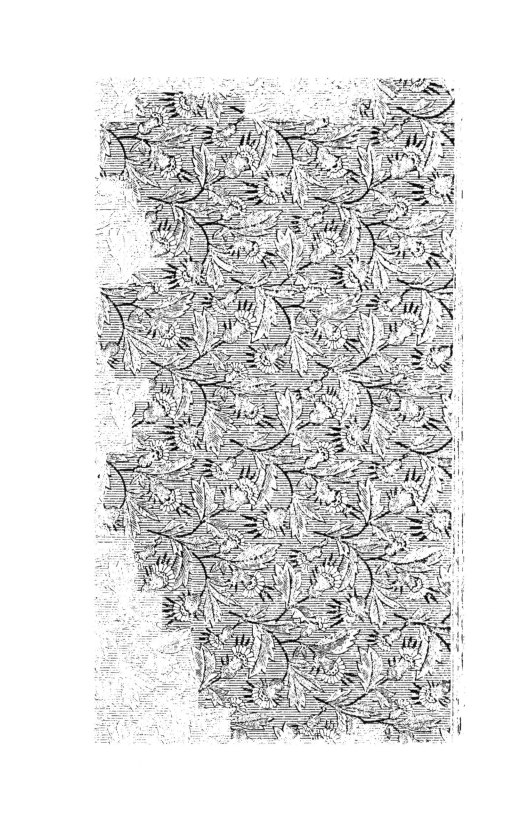

9 9.

# REPERTORY
# OF THE SYMPTOMS

OF

# RHEUMATISM, SCIATICA,

## ET CETERA.

BY

ALFRED PULFORD, M. D.

*All forms of substance are but gases in various stages of density; Divine power being invisible, lays latent in all objects, organic or inorganic, hence the triumph of Homœopathic medication.*

TIFFIN, OHIO:
B. B. KRAMMES, PUBLISHER.

# 16321

# PREFACE.

---

In vain has been the search for a work on Rheumatism that was at once up-to-date, available and reliable, but so far have not been able to find one, and like Bell with his immortal work on Diarrhœa, etc., have gathered together in the past twelve years reliable and verified symptoms and put them in convenient form, but as my script is almost unreadable, concluded to print the MSS. and give my friends the benefit, for which reason this work appears among you.

.The publication of this work was offered to Boericke and Tafel, but as they already had a ten year old work on hand they hardly felt like printing another one, and I inferred from this that there would not be any other work published on Rheumatism as long as a copy of the ten year old edition could be sold.

Rheumatism, while a very prevalent disease, seems to me to have been a very much neglected subject as far as works go. That there is and has been a demand for works on this subject is evinced by the large number of subscriptions already received for this little book.

It is the sincere wish of the compiler of this Repertory that it may prove as great a convenience to his fellow physicians as it has to himself.

Dr. A. Pulford.

*Tiffin, Ohio, Aug. 15, 1898.*

# INTRODUCTION.

In compiling this Repertory the object has been to arrange and classify groups and conditions of symptoms in such a manner that they may be readily available. In carrying out the plan laid out it was deemed unnecessary to give a list of remedies, but will suffice to say that all remedies, where there is any doubt as to their identity, have been spelled sufficient to reveal themselves. It may be well to state here, however, that the small letter (p) in Calc. p. stands for "phos." as it also does in Kali p., etc., the letter "c" stands for "carb.", "ac." for acid, "m" for mur. except in metallic substances. Remedies having several adjectives, like Kali phos., permang., Calc. phos., pic., etc. will be found to have all others spelled out except the abbreviation "phos."

When reading under a subject, say pain, a reference to any other subject under pain would refer you by the word beginning with a small letter, should the word begin with a capital it will refer you to a subject other than pain. The abbreviations "alt." and "Esp." have been used in place of "alternation" and "especially." Profuse references have been made in order to avoid too much repetition.

The crescendo and diminuendo marks have been used throughout the work to express aggravation and amelioration, etc.

In cases where many remedies have been stated, the more important ones have been emphasized; where only one or two are named it has not been deemed necessary to follow out this plan, so that should you find a remedy not in capitals or italics do not pass it by as unimportant, for it may be very important.

A. PULFORD, M. D.

*Tiffin, Ohio.*

# AGGRAVATIONS.

ACIDS: Brom.

AIR, cool or cold: Caust., Cist., Dulc., Phos., *Rhus;* **Reverse**:
     PULS.

> Open: *Rhus*, SIL.; **Reverse**: Acon., Asa., Bry.,
>      *Cyc.*, Dios., Lyc., Mez.,Natr.s.,Pet.,
>      Plat., PULS.

Exposure to: Hep.

Least draught of: Bell.

Walking in open: Agar.

AFTERNOON until midnight: Bell.

ALONE, when: Phos., Stram.

ANKLES, in: Agar.

A. M.: Agar., *Aloe*, *Ars.*, Bov., *Bry.*, Dios., Ferr., *Hep.*,
     *Kali c.*, Lyc., Mangan., NUX, Puls., Sep.,
     Staph., SULF.; **Reverse**: Aur.

1, after: Ars., *Lyc.*

2: Ars., *Lyc.*, *Nux.*

  And 4: *Nux.*

3: Caul., KALI C., *Nux*, Sep., Verat.

  To 5: Sep.

4: Nux.

5: *Aloe*, Sep., SULF.

And P.M.: SEP., Sulf.

     In bed: Sulf.

     Noon: Arg. nit.

Early: NUX.

In and toward: Ferr.

  Bed: Mangan., Puls., Staph., *Sulf.*

On rising: Lyc.

Towards: ARS., Bov., *Kali c.*, Nux, LYC., Rhus,
     Thuya.

BACK: See Lying.

BATH, after a: Ant. c.

BED, covering intolerable: *Led.*, Sulf.; **Reverse:** *Agar.*

> Driving one out of: *Ferr.*, Puls.
>
> Heat of, which is intolerable: Apis, *Led.*, Merc., Verat.; **Reverse:** *Agar.*
>
> In: Arn., *Ferr.*, Kali bi., *Led.*, *Merc.*, *Rhus*, Verat.; **Reverse:** *Agar.*, *Caust.*
>
> Lying in, and getting warm in: Arn.; **Reverse:** *Agar.*
>
> Mornings in: Mangan., Puls., Staph., SULF.
>
> Nights in: Amm. m., FERR., *Mag.*, *Merc.*, Nux, RHUS, *Sang.*, Verat.
>
> Turning in: Arn., *Nux*, Zinc. ox.
> > Must sit up first: *Nux.*
>
> Warm, getting in: Arn., Sulf.
> > And lying in: Arn.; **Reverse:** *Agar.*, *Caust.*

BENDING backward: Rhus; **Reverse:** Bell.

BLOWING nose: Calc. p.

BREAKFAST, after: Phos.

> See also Eating.

COFFEE, after: Caul., *Ign.*

COLD: Amm. c., *Calc.*, Cist., Graph., Kali c., RHUS, SIL.; **Reverse:** PULS.

> After taking: Cham.
>
> Air: Cist., RHUS; **Reverse:** PULS.
>
> Drinks: Ant. c.; **Reverse:** Phos., PULS.
>
> Open air: SIL.; **Reverse:** PULS.
>
> Water externally: Ant. c., Phos., Sulf.
> > Internally: Ant. c., Lyc.; **Reverse:** Phos., Puls.
> > And externally: Ant. c.
>
> When becoming: Graph.
>
> See also Weather.

COMBING hair: Rhus.

CONTACT or motion, no<or>by: Bell.

COUGHING: Tell.

COVERED, from being: Ferr., *Led.*, Lyc., Sulf.; **Reverse:** Agar., Caust., Hep., Nux, Rhus, *Sil.*

DAMPNESS: Dulc., Natr.s., Phyt., Rhod., Sarsap.

DANCING: Alum.

DARK, in the: Stram.; **Reverse:** Phos.

DAY, only during: Col.

> Every other: *Ars.*, CHIN.S., *Ferr.*, Lyc.

DINNER, after: Zinc.

> See also Eating.

DRAWING up limbs: Rhus; **Reverse:** Sulf.

DRINKS, cold: Ant. c., Ars.; **Reverse:** *Phos., Puls.*

Hot: Phos.; **Reverse:** Lyc.

EATING, after: Cann. s., Indigo, NUX, Phos., Sep., Zinc.

Breakfast: Phos.

Cold food: Puls.; **Reverse:** Phos.

Dinner: Zinc.

Fat food: *Cyc.*, PULS.

Supper: Iris.

Warm food: Phos.; **Reverse:** Puls.

EMISSIONS, after: Cobalt.

ERUPTIONS, from suppression of cutaneous: Phos. ac., *Psor., Sulf.*

EVENINGS: Acon., Bry., Caust., Col., Colch., Fagop., Hell., *Iod.*, Iris, Led., Lyc., MERC., Mez., *Nit ac.*, Oleand., Phos., Plat., Plumb., PULS., RHUS, Sticta, Sulf., Zinc.

And night: Acon., Arn., ARS., Bell., Bry., *Cham.*, China, Dulc., Graph., *Hep.*, MERC., Mez., *Phos., Puls.*, Sticta.

2 to 9 P. M.: Syphil.

And all night: Syph.

3 P. M.: Apis, Chin. s.

After: Bell.

4 to 6 P. M.: *Carbo v.*

8 P. M.: LYC.

5 P. M.: Apis.

11 P. M.: Bell.

Until: Lyc.

Midnight: Led., Phos., Puls.

EVERY third week: Mag. c.

See also Day.

EXERTION, bodily: Bell., Sulf.

Mental: NUX.

Slightest: Natr. c.

FLEXING leg on abdomen: Col.; **Reverse:** Kali bi.

FOODS, cold: Puls.; **Reverse:** Phos.

Fat: Cyc., PULS.

Warm: Phos.

HANGING limb out of bed: Vipera; **Reverse:** Verat.

HEAT: Ant. c., Bell., Col., Glon., *Lyc.*, MERC., PULS., SEC., Verat.; **Reverse:** Ars., *Caust.*, Colch., HEP., MAG., RHUS, SIL., Sulf.

HEAT: Applied to parts: Lyc., *Sec.;* **Reverse:** Hep., Mag., Rhus, etc.

Of bed: Led., Verat.; **Reverse:** Agar.

Sun: Ant. c., Bell., Glon.

INSPIRATION, deep: Acon., Aeth., Bry., Fagop., Spig.

INTERMITTENTLY: Ign.

JAR, least: Salycil. ac.

JOINTS: Dros., Kali bi., Magnol., Puls.

Smaller: Act. s., Kali bi.

Larger: Bry.

KNEES, r.: Chel.

LAUGHING: Tell.

L. side: Cann. i., Cim., Crot. t., Ferr., Hydrast., LACH., *Merc. bin., Rhus*, Stann., Stram., Sulf.

LIFTING anything, attempting to: Curare.

LIFTING: *Calc. p.*, Nux, Rhus.

LIMB hanging down: Calc.; **Reverse:** *Bell.*, Verat.

Straightening out: Val.; **Reverse:** Rhus.

LYING: Acon., Aeth., AMM. M., Ars., Berb., Bry., Carbo an., *Ferr.*, Gossyp., Kali bi., Merc., Natr. s., Puls., RHUS, Sil., Spig., Sulf., Tell.

Down at night: *Ars.*, Berb., FERR., Kali bi., RHUS, Tell.

During day: *Merc. bin.*

On affected side: Bry., Kali i., Sil., Tell.; **Reverse:** Bry., Puls.

Back: Amm. m., Gossyp., Phos., Puls., Spig.; **Reverse:** Calc., Convall., Natr. m.

L. side: Natr. s., Puls.; **Reverse:** Bry., Merc.

Painful side: Hep., Kali i., Nux m., Sil., Tell.; **Reverse:** Bry., Puls.

Painless side: Puls.

R. side: Bry., Merc.; **Reverse:** Natr. s., Phos., Puls., Sulf.

Sitting and: Amm. m., Berb., Ferr., Kali bi., Merc., Rhus.; **Reverse:** BRY.

Standing and: Kali bi., Rhus.

Standing and: Carbo an., Rhus, Sulf.

Still: RHUS; **Reverse:** *Bry.*, Col., DIOS.

Walking and: Bry., Carbo an., Natr. s., Puls., Rhus, Sil., Sulf.; **Reverse:** Puls.

MEALS, after: Indigo.

See also Eating.

MENSES, at: Mag. c.

Before: Sep.

During: Graph., Mag. c.

And after: Graph.

MENTAL effort: NUX.

MERCURY, after: Hep., Nit. ac., Phyt., Sarsap., Sil.

MIDNIGHT, after: ARS., Merc., *Rhus*, Sulf., Thuya.

Afternoon until: Bell.

Before: Bry., Rhus.

Evening until: Led., Phos., *Puls.*

MOON, during full: Calc., Sulf.

New: Canst., SIL.

Or near full: Calc.

MORNING: See A. M.

MOTION: Acon., *Act. s.*, BRY., Calc., Caust., CHINA, Cina, Col., DIOS., *Ferr. p.*, Form., Iris, Kali c., Led., Phyt., Ox. ac., Puls., Ran. bulb., Rhus, Senec., SIL., Spig., Staph., Sulf.

And contact: *Act. s., Bry., China.*

No<or> from: Bell.

Pressure: Col., Phyt.

As if pains would be, from, but are not: Calc. p.

Effort at, causes cold perspiration and retching: Ant. t.

Esp. raising arm: Iris.

From any, of arms or lying on back: Spig.

Moderate, not altered by violent: Iris.

No>at rest: Iris.

Nor<from contact or: Bell.

Not<by: Cina.

On commencement of: Lyc., *Puls.*, RHUS, Sep.

Slightest: *Arn.*, Bell., BRY., CHINA, *Cim.*, DIOS., Guiac., Mangan., SALYCIL. AC., Sang.

Touch and: Bell., Hep., Mez., Sabin., Staph.

Turning in bed: Arn., Nux, Zinc. ox.

Violent: Ruta; **Reverse:** Niccol.

Yet not>lying down: Ran. bulb.

See also Walking.

MUSCULAR part of thighs: Plumb.

NEITHER<nor>by, or contact: Bell.

Rest: Cann. i., Rhus.

NO<: Cann. i., Rhus.
  While walking: Rhus; **Reverse:** Bry.

NIGHT: ARS., Aur., Bell., *Cham.*, Coff., *Ferr., Iod.*,
  Ign., Kali bi. and i., Led., Lyc., *Mag.*,
  Mangan., MERC., Mez., *Nit.ac.*, Nitrum.,
  *Phos. ac.*, Phyt., Plumb., *Puls.*, Rhod.,
  RHUS, Salycil. ac., *Sang.*, Sil., Sticta,
  Sulf., Zinc. met. and ox.

  And evening: See Evening.
  Driving one out of bed: FERR.
  In bed: See Bed.
  Toward: China, Colch., Led., Merc., Phos., *Puls.*
  With fever and restlessness: Mag. c.

OUT doors: Bell.; **Reverse:** Mez., Natr. s., PULS.

PERSPIRING, while: *Lach.*, MERC., Opi., TILIA;
  **Reverse:** Gels., NATR. M., Nux.

P. M.: See Evening.

PRESSING at stool: Carbo an., Nux, Tell.

PRESSURE: Acon., Caps., CHINA, Cina, Col., *Hep.*,
  *Kali bi.*, Pip. m., *Sil ;* **Reverse:** COL.,
  Stann.

  External: Cina, Hep., Col., Stann.

POULTICES, hot: LYC.; **Reverse:** Rhus.
  Wet: Sulf.; **Reverse:** Nux. m.

RAISING arm: *Alum.*, Ferr., Hyos., *Iris*, Led., Mag. c.,
  RHUS, Sang.
  Upward and backward: *Calc.*, RHUS.

REST: *Calc.*, Col., Dulc., Euphorb., Indigo, Kali p., *Merc.
  bin.*, RHUS, Staph., Sep., Sulf.; **Reverse:**
  BRY.. Dios.

  After: *Calc.*, *Kali p.*, RHUS.
  At: Euphorb., *Indigo*, RHUS.
  During: Staph.; **Reverse:** BRY., MERC.

RIDING in a carriage: *Coccul.*, Nux m., Pet.; **Reverse:**
  Graph., Nit. ac.
  Or train: *Coccul.*, Pet.

R. SIDE: Caust., CHEL., *Col.*, LYC., *Phyt.*, Tell., Val.
  Knee: Chel.
  To l.: Apis, Lach., LYC.

RISING: *Aesc.*, Aloe, Ant. c., Arg. nit., Berb., Caust..
  *Kali p.*, LACH., Lyc., Nit. ac., Phos.,
  Puls., RHUS, SIL., Zinc.
  Early on: Thuya; **Reverse:** Cham.

  From a seat or chair: Anac., Ant. c., Arg. nit.,
  Berb., Caust., *Kali p.*, LACH., Lyc.,
  Nit. ac., Phos., Puls., *Rhus*, SIL.,
  Zinc.
  Stooping: *Aesc.*, RHUS, Zinc.

RISING, from, must sit still: LACH.

Or standing erect: Aesc., Aloe.

ROOM, cool: *Bell.*, Rhus; **Reverse**: PULS., Sabina.

Warm: PULS., Sabina.

SEWING: Ran. bulb., Zinc.

Long continued: Ran. bulb.

SIDE not lain on: Rhus.

See also Lying, L., R.

SITTING: Amm. m., Bell., Berb., Cobalt., Col., Dig., Dios., Euphorb., Ferr., *Kali bi.*, LACH., *Mag. m.*, Merc., Pet., RHUS, Tongo, Val., Verat., Zinc.

Cannot rise after: Bell., LACH.

Must sit still: LACH.

Must be careful not to press the limbs while: Col.

Standing and: Kali bi., Rhus, Val., Verat.

Walking and: Val.

Still: RHUS, Zinc.; **Reverse**: *Acon., Bry.,* DIOS.

Up: Dios., Mag. m.; **Reverse**: Verat.

Walking or: Col., Mag. m., Zinc.; **Reverse**: Verat.

See also Lying.

SLEEP, after: LACH.; **Reverse**: Phos.

Broken: NUX.

During: Cham.; **Reverse**: Crot. t.

SNEEZING: Aeth.

SPRING: See Summer.

STAIRS, ascending: Ars., Calc., COCA.

Descending: Borax, Stann.

STANDING: Agar., AESC., Carbo an., *Kali bi.*, KALI C., Rhus, SUL., Thuya, *Val.*, Verat.

And sitting: Kali bi., Rhus, Sulf., Val., Verat.

Walking: AESC., Agar., Carbo an., KALI C., Sulf., Thuya, Val.

Or walking: Aesc., Ign.

Sitting or walking: Sulf., Val.

Thigh feels as if it would break off when: Val.

See also Lying.

STEPPING heavily on ground: Rhus.

STIMULANTS: Acon., ANT. C., Ars., Glon., Ign., Lyc., Nux, Sil., Zinc.

Brandy: Ign.

On taking: Acon.

STIMULANTS: Spirituous: Nux m.
>    Wine: Acon., ANT. C., Ars., Glon., Lyc., Nux, Sil.,
>       ZINC.
>    Sour: ANT. C.

STOOL, during hard: Nux.
>    On pressing at: Carbo an., Nux, Tell.

STOOPING: *Aesc.*, Cic., Cim., Lith. c., RHUS, *Sulf.*,
>       Zinc.
>    Forward: *Aesc.*, Cim.
>    On rising from: Aesc., RHUS, Zinc.

STORM, before a: Rhod.
>    Easterly: Canst.
>    Thunder, before a: Petr.
>       During a: Natr. c., Phos.

STRAIGHTENING out limb: Val.; **Reverse**: Rhus.

SUMMER and spring with cool days and nights: Kali bi.

SWEAT, during: Cham.; **Reverse**: NATR. M.

SWEATING, while: Lach., Merc., Tilia.

SYPHILIS: Phyt., Sarsap.

TALKING: Bell.

THINKING of troubles: Bar. c.. Caust., *Ox. ac.*, *Pip. m.*;
>       **Reverse**: Camph., Hell.

THUNDER: See Storm.

TOBACCO, chewing: Ars., Nux, Plant.
>    Smoking: Ign.

TOUCH: Agnus, *Arn.*, Bell., CHINA, *Colch.*, Cup., Hep.,
>       Mangan., Nit. ac., Staph., Sulf.; **Reverse**:
>       Bry.
>    Fears the possibility of: ARN., CHINA, *Colch.*
>    Or motion: Sabina.

TURNING in bed: Arn., Nux, Zinc. ox.
>       Must sit up before: NUX.
>    Trunk: Thuya.

UTERINE pains: Ambra.

WALKING: AESC., Agar., Anac., BRY., Carbo an.
>       and v., Chel., Cim., Col., Colch., Ferr.,
>       *Graph.*, Hep., Hydrast., KALI C., Mag.
>       m., Natr. s., Nux, Phos., Plumb., Rhus,
>       Sabin., Sil., SULF., Thuya, *Val.*, *Zinc.*
>    After: Natr. s., Phos.
>    Fatigues: Graph., Plumb.
>    In open air: Agar., Sil., Zinc.
>       Wind: Bell.
>    See also Lying, Sitting, Standing.

WARM, on becoming: LED., Sil.

 Getting, in bed: Merc., Sulf.; **Reverse**: Agar., Canst.

 Room, in: PULS., Sabin.; **Reverse**: Bell.

WARMTH: Bry., *Ferr.*, Kali s., LED., *Lyc.*, *Merc.*, Phos., PULS., Thuya, Verat.

 See also Bed.

WASHING: Nit. ac., Phos., Sep., *Sulf.*

 Hands: *Phos.*

 In water: Phos., Sep., *Sulf.*

WATER: Ant. c., Calc., Nit. ac., *Phos.*, Puls., Rhus, *Sulf.*

 Cold, internally and externally: Ant. c.

 Bathing in: Ant. c.

 Wetting feet in: Puls., Tarent.

  Or hands in: Tarent.

 Working or standing in: CALC., Rhus.

 See also washing.

WEATHER, at every change of: Bry., Carbo v., Mangan., Phos., Rhod., Sil., Verat.

 Change of, esp. damp: Calc., Dulc.; Ran. bulb.

 Changing from warm to cold: Dulc

 Cold: *Calc.*, Dulc., *Ign.*, Merc., Nux m., Phos., Phyt., Rhod., RHUS, Sil., Verat., Viola t.

  Damp: Calc., *Dulc.*, Merc., Phos., Phyt., Rhod., Verat.

 Damp: China, DULC., Natr. s., Phyt., Ran. bulb., RHUS.

 Hot: *Kali bi.*, Lathyrus, Phos., Puls., Xanth.; **Reverse**: Calc. p., IGN., Rhus.

 Rainy: *Rhod.*: See Damp.

 Rough: *Rhod.*, Viola t.

 Wet: Agar., Lathyrus, Nux m., Phos., Sil.

 Windy: Rhod., Viola t.

WET: SIL., Sulf.

WETTING feet: Puls.

 Hands: Phos.

WINE: See Stimulants.

WINTER: *Ign.*, *Rhus.*

WRITING: Merc. iod., Ran. bulb., *Zinc.*

WRISTS and hands: Curare.

# AMELIORATIONS.

AIR, from open: Acon., PULS.
    Cool: PULS.
    Open: Acon., Asa., Bry., *Cyc.*, Dios., *Lyc.*, Mez.,
        Natr. s., Pet., Plat., PULS:
    Warm: Pet.
APPLICATIONS, cold: Apis, Fluo. ac., Puls.
        Hot: China, Rhus.
        Dry: Rhus.
        Moist: Nux m.
        Warm external: *Ars.*, Col., Colch., HEP.,
          MAG., *Rhus*, SIL.
BED, while in: Canst.
    Being warm in: Agar.
    Hanging limb out of: Verat.
BENDING backward: Bell., *Rhus.*
    Double: COL.
    Inward: Bell.
    Leg: Kali bi.
CHANGE of position: Arn., Ox. ac., PULS., *Rhus.*
        Bed or couch on which he lies feels too
          hard: ARN.
        For a few moments: Rhus.
COLD applications: Apis, Fluo. ac., Puls.
    Drinks, esp. water: *Puls.*
    Food, eating: Phos.
    External: Puls., Thuya.
COOL place: Puls.
DARK, in: Phos.
DAYLIGHT approaches, as: Syphil.
DRINKS, cold: Phos., Puls.
    Hot: Lyc.
EATING cold food: Phos.
ELEVATING knee: Calc.
EVENING, towards: Kali bi. and c.
    Until: Lyc.

EXCITEMENT, pleasant: Kali p., *Pip. m.*

FASTING, while: Cham.

FLATUS, passing: Alum., Col.

FLEXING leg: Kali bi.

HANDS of another person: Asa.

HANGING limb out of bed: Verat.

HEAT: *Ars.*, Caust., Colch., HEP., MAG., RHUS, *Sil.*, Sulf.

> Dry: Rhus.
> External: Ars.
> Moist: Nux m.

KEEPING heels higher than head: Phyt.

'KNEES, elevating: Calc.

LIGHT, bright: Stram.

LIMBS, drawing up: Sulf.

> Elevating knee: Calc.
> Hanging down: *Bell.*, Verat.
> Stretching out: Rhus.

LYING: AMM.M., Anac., *Bry.*, Col., Convall., Dios., Natr. m., Nux, Puls.

> Down: Anac., Calc. p., AMM. M., Merc.
>> Not>: Ran. bulb.
> On affected side: Bry., Puls.
>> Back: Bry., *Calc.*, Convall., Lyc., NATR. M., Puls., Sang.
>> R. side: Phos., Sulf.
>> Side: Puls.
>> Something hard: Natr. m.
>> Well side: Nux.
> Still: *Bry.*, Col., *Dios.*
>> Perfectly: *Dios.*
> Walking or: Puls.

MORNING: Aur. met.

MOTION: Acon., Aloe, *Ars.*, *Calc.*, Caps., Caust., Dios., *Eup. perf.*, *Ferr.*, Kali c. and iod., Menyanth., Phos. ac., Cina, *Puls.*, Rhod., RHUS, Ruta, Senec., Staph., Sulf., Tongo, Zinc.

> Continued: Caps., *Rhus*, Ruta.
> During: Sulf.
> From: Staph.
> Of feet: Caust., Zinc.

MOTION or contact, no>or<from: Bell.

    Slow: Ferr., Puls.

    Violent: Niccol.

MOVING affected parts: RHUS.

NEITHER>nor<: Bell., *Cann. i.*, Rhus.

            By, motion or contact: Bell.

                   Rest: Rhus.

NO> from sweat: Lach., Merc. corr.

OUT doors: Mez., Natr. s., PULS.

PERSPIRING: Apis, Bell., Cham., Graph., NATR. M., Nux.

    After: Bell., Cham., Graph.

    While: Gels., NATR. M., Nux.

PRESSING against something hard: Natr. m., Rhus.

    On parts: Bell., Puls., Rhus.

PRESSURE: *China*, COL., Form., Natr. m., Pip. m., Puls., Stann.

    Firm: China, Col.

    Hard: COL.

    Nightly pains: Phos. ac.

    Sometimes: Phos. ac.

REST: BRY., Col., *Dios.*, Hep., Merc., Sep.

    When at: Merc.

RIDING in a carriage: Graph., Nit. ac.

RISING, after: Eup. perf., Sulf.

    On: Cham.

ROOM, cool: PULS.

    Warm: Bell.

RUBBING: Amm. m., Phos.

SEASON, cool: Puls.

    Warm: Calc. p., IGN , *Rhus.*

SITTING still: Acon., Bry.

    Up: Verat.

    Walking or: Verat.

SLEEP, after: Phos.

    During: Crot. t.

    Unbroken: Nux.

STANDING: Ant. c., Arg. nit., Bell., Thuya.

SUMMER: Calc. p., IGN., Rhus.

SUPPURATION: Stram.

SWEAT: See Perspiration.

THINKING of symptoms: Camph., Hell.

THROWING shoulders back and chest forward: Badiago.

TIGHT bandaging: Trill.

TOUCH: Bry.

UNCOVERING: Led., Lyc., Puls., Sulf.

URINATING: Lyc.

WALKING: Aloe, Ant. c., Arg. nit., Bell., Cann. s., *Ferr.*, Indigo, *Kali bi.*, MERC., Puls., RHUS, Staph., Sulf., Thuya, *Val.*, Verat.

    About, slowly: FERR., *Puls.*, Verat.

WARM air: Pet.

    Applications: Ars., Rhus.

        External: Rhus.

    Being, in bed: Agar.

    Room: Bell.

    Season: Calc. p., IGN., Rhus.

    Wraps: *Ars.*, *Atrop.*, Bell., Bry., Hep., Sec., SIL.

WARMTH: *Ars.*, Bell., Caust., Col., *Hep.*, Kali s., Lyc., MAG., Merc., RHUS, Sec., SIL., Sulf.

    Of bed: Caust., Col.

WATER, cold applications of: Apis, Fluo. ac.

    Hot applications of: Nux m.

WEATHER, cold: PULS.

    Dry: Nux m., Sulf.

    Hot: Calc. p., IGN., Rhus.

WRAPS: See Warm.

# NECK.

---

ACHING: Onos., Sep.

    Dull: Onos.

    In back of: Sep.

ACROMION, dull, intermittent pressure as from a heavy load on r. side of N. and l. A.: Anac.

AIR, stiffness of neck from cold: Dulc.

    See also Pain rheumatic.

BEATING in muscles of N.: Cyc.

BROKEN, sensation as if N. were: Chel.

BRUISED feeling and stiffness in l. side of N., extending to l. shoulder, ear and back, <lying, >motion: Acon.

    See also Pain bruised.

CHEST: Tearing in side of N. alt. with same in C.: Amm. m.

CLAVICLE: See Pain in.

COLD, neuralgia due to C. or nervous shock, N. stiff, < 3 A. M. after eating and touch: Nux.

    Stiff N. from, air: Dulc.

CONTRACTION of r. sterno-cleido-mastoid, no pain or inflammation: Bell.

CONSTRICTION of N., Iod.

CRACKING in: Chel., Oleum. an.

        Vertebrae with stiffness on moving N.: Chel.

CRAMPS of muscles, and spasmodic drawing backward of head: *Cic.*, Cim.

DRAWING in muscles of N.: Acon.

    See also Cramps and Pain drawing.

ENLARGEMENT of glands: Bar., Calc., Carbo v., Phyt., Still.

        N.: Cup.

EMACIATED and shrunken: Sarsap.

    Greatly: Calc. p., *Natr. m.*, Sarsap.

FEET: See Pain rheumatic.

GLANDS enlarged: Bar., Calc., Carbo v., Phyt., Still.

> Indurated: *Arg. n.*, Calc. fluo., Con.
>
> Sore with pain under l. scapula (Chel. r.): Ail.
>
> Swollen: Iod.
>
> > Of N. and occiput: Bar., Calc., Carbo v.
>
> See also Pain jerking.

HAMMER; sensation in nape as if struck by a: Bell.

HEAD drawn to l. side: *Lachn.*, Nux.

> Dullness of H. and stiff N. from least draught of air: Calc. p.
>
> Feels as if N. would not support H.: Acon.
>
> Heaviness of H., with weakness of cervical and dorsal muscles: Verat.

HEAD; N. too weak to support the: Calc. p., Natr. m.

> > > It falls from side to side: Calc. p.
>
> Retraction of H. and N.: Cim.
>
> Rigidity of muscles of N., with a great deal of pain and inability to turn H.: Tarent. H.
>
> Sinks forward with weakness of nape of N.: Plat.
>
> Spasmodic drawing backward of H., with spasms and cramps in N.: Cic.
>
> Stiffness of N. from getting H. wet: Bell., Bry., Calc.
>
> > On moving H. (Bry.), with painfulness on deep breathing: Chel.
>
> See also Pain.

HEADACHE extends to nape of N.: Lyc.

> With stiffness of nape of N.: Sil.

HIPS; Bruised sensation in nape, thighs and: Phos. ac.

HEAVINESS and stiffness as from a load on nape, with painful tension: Vinca m.

> Of head with weakness of cervical and dorsal muscles: Verat. a.
>
> Stiffness and weariness, with painful tension as from a load: Vinca m.
>
> With tension of nape of N.: Chel.
>
> See also Pain.

INVOLUNTARY stretching of N.: Lyc.

JERKING motion in N.: Canst.

> See Pain tearing.

LAMENESS of N.: Natr. c.

> And weariness: *Aesc.*, Zinc.

LOAD; Dull intermittent pressure as from a heavy, on r. side of N.: Anac.

Weariness of nape as from a heavy: Paris.

Stiffness and tension with painful heaviness as from a: Vinca m.

LOSS of power in nape of N.: Nit. ac.

MUSCLES of back and N. rigid: Caul.

So painful that motion is impossible: Tarent. H.

MOTION jerking in N.: Caust.

NAPE; Aching in: Cann. i., Naja, Rhus.

Boring and stiffness in: Psor.

Bruised sensation in, hips and thighs: Phos. ac.

Drawing: Chel., Natr. c., *Pet.*, Stram., Sulf.

Very painful distressing, in, extending to occiput: Pet.

Glands of, and occiput swollen: Bar.

Greatly constricted: Nux m.

Head, spasmodic drawing backward of, with spasms and cramps of muscles of N.: Cic.

Sinks forward with weakness of N.: Plat.

Stiffness of muscles of N. on moving H.: Col. Dulc.

Headache with stiffness of N.: Sil.

Heaviness and stiffness as from a load, with painful tension: Vinca m.

Tension of muscles: Chel.

In: Pet.

Or Pain: Pet.

Hammer, sensation in, as if struck by a: Bell.

Hips, bruised sensation in N. and: Phos. ac.

Load, stiffness and heaviness as from a: with painful tension: Vinca m.

Weariness as from a heavy: Paris.

Loss of power of N.: Nit. ac.

Occiput, glands of N. and, swollen: Bar. c. and m.

Very painful distressing drawing in N. extends to: Pet.

Pain; Aching: Cann. i., Naja, Rhus.

Beating in N. and occiput, >after rising: Eup. perf.

Distressing, in N. and occiput: Aeth.

Drawing in N.: Natr. c., *Pet.*

Rheumatic, from N.: Chel.

Extends to head from N.: Carbo v.

NAPE; Pain: In N. alt. with violent pain and heaviness, in head: Hyos.

As if head had been lying in an uncomfortable position: Dulc.

With spasmodic rigidity, coming from smaller joints: Caul.

Rheumatic: *Puls.*, Staph.

With weariness in feet: Puls.

Saddle, as from a, across N.: Thuya.

Sticking: Natr. m. and s., Puls.

Stiff, and in external cervical muscles: Mez.

Tearing, by paroxysms, in evening: Nux.

Tensive in N. and in occiput, while writing: *Lyc.*. Zinc.

Weight or, in: Pet.

Painful: Aeth., Aesc., Carbo v., Caul., Chel., Con., Dros., Dulc., Eup., Mez., Nux, *Pet.* *Puls.*, Staph.

Paralyzed as if: Rhus.

Rheumatism: Hell., Mag. c., Merc.

Saddle, pain from a, across: Thuya.

Sensation as if a load on N.. with paralyzed S. in limbs on Walking: Rhus.

N. was struck by a hammer: Bell.

Of stiffness in N. and in neck, l. side, extending into ear: Thuya.

Sensitive to external impressions: Lach.

Spasms and cramps in muscles of N. and spasmodic drawing backward of head and painful tension on inner surface of scapula: Cic.

Sticking in: Natr. m., *Puls.*

At night: Natr. m.

Stiffness and heaviness as from a load, with painful tension: Vinca m.

Of: *Acon.*, Agar., *Bell.*, *Bry.*, Calc. p., Canst., *Chel.*, Col., *Dulc.*, *Ferr.p.*, Graph., Ign., Kali c., *Lachn.*, Nitr. ac., Nux, *Phos.*, *Rhus*, Sil., *Sulf.*, *Thuy.*

In morning; in bed: Kali c.

Muscles on moving head: Col., Dulc.

Rheumatic: Rhus.

Sensation of, in N. and neck, l. side, extending into ear: Thuya.

NAPE; Stiffness, torticollis, r. side, muscles contracted and painful swelling and stiffness: Bell., Bry.

With headache: Sil.

Heaviness in N.: Ginseng.

Tearing in N.: Kalm.

Tension, painful, with stiffness and heaviness as from a load: Vinca m.

Torticollis, r. side, muscles contracted or painful swelling and stiffness: Bell., Bry.

Walking, sensation as of a load on N. with paralyzed feeling in limbs on: Rhus.

Weakness of N., head sinks forward: Plat.

Weariness evenings and while writing: Lyc., Zinc.

Weary as from a heavy load: Paris.

Writing: See Pain tensive and Weariness.

NEURALGIA cervico - brachial, N., < early A. M., after eating and from touch, due to cold and nervous shock: Nux.

PAIN; Aching: Onos., Sep.

Dull: Onos.

In back of: Sep.

Air, rheumatic, from slightest of, causing stiffness of N. and dullness of head: Calc. p.

And stiffness of upper dorsal and cervical muscles: Zinc.

Arm, from N. down r. to little finger: Kalm.

Beaten, as if: Zinc.

Bruised, in back of N.: *Acon.*, Dig., Hep.

Clavicle, in r. cervical muscles and: Chel., (Magnol.).

Cramplike: Calc. p.

Darting, sticking: Ferrum.

Drawing in muscles of N. Acon.

R. side of N.: Sulf.

Rheumatic: Chel., Cyc.

Dull, in back of N.: Fagop.

Extends from shoulder to N. Apis.

Finger: See Arm.

From back of head to forehead: Sang., Sil., Spig.

Forehead to back of N.: Onos.

N. down r. arm to little finger: Kalm.

Extending to head: Carbo v.

In head and N. intense with inflammatory rheumatism of small joints: Sticta.

PAIN in N. and occiput, with screaming: Natr. s.

On turning head: Bry., Calc., Rhus.

R. cervical muscles and r. clavicle (Magnol.) Chel.

Insupportable, on looking up: Form.

Jerking, tearing, in r. cervical glands: Caps.

Lacerating, in posterior cervical muscles: Calc., caust.

N. tender to touch with: Kalm.

On turning head: *Bry.*, *Calc.*, Rhus.

Paralyzed: Chel.

Rheumatic: Acon., Calc. p., China, Cham., *Cim.*, Clem., Dulc.

From slightest draft of air, causing stiffness of N. and dullness of head: Calc. p.

In N. and muscles of back, with stiffness and contraction: China, *Cim.*, Clem., Dulc.

Violent: Graph.

Severe, dull: Dros.

In cervical region: Lach.

Sticking in nape: Natr., Puls.

Stiff, in moving cervical muscles and yawning: Coccul.

Tearing: Kali c., Nux, Oleand., Phos., Zinc.

On motion: Kali c.

Tensive, and pressure: Bell., Carbo v.

Extending to N.: Crotal h.

In nape: Lyc.

Violent, drawing in l. cervical muscles<motion: Col.

Terrible: Pic. ac.

PAINFUL, all muscles of N. so, that motion is impossible: Tarent H.

Muscles of N. Hep.

♦ Nape: Aesc., Chel., *Pet.*, *Puls.*

` Stiffness: Merc., *Mez.*, Natr. s.

And tension: Colch., Dig.

PARALYZED, muscles of nape seem: Verat.

PARALYSIS: Colch., Plumb.

Of cervical muscles: *Plumb.*

PRESSURE, dull intermittent, as from a heavy load on r. side of N. and l. acromion: Anac.

See also Pain tensive.

RETRACTION of head and N. Cim.

RHEUMATIC stiffness: Rhus, Verat.

    Stitches: Apis.

RIGIDITY of muscles: Stram.

               With great pain and inability
                     to turn head: Tarent. H.

SENSATION as if nape were struck with a hammer:
                             Bell.

          N. were broken: Chel.

      Of a load on N. and of paralyzed limbs
                     on walking: Rhus.

          Stiffness in nape and l. side, extending
                     into ear: Thuya.

          Weakness: Caps.

SHAKES and trembles: Carbo v.

SHARP twisting in back of N.: Dros.

SHRUNKEN, N. greatly emaciated and: Sarsap.

SLENDER, too, to support the head: Calc. p., Natr.m.

SPASMS and cramps in N. with spasmodic drawing
                  backward of the head: Cic.

SPRAINED sensation: Agar.

STICKING in: Lach.

STIFF and sore: Ars., Fagop., Ferr.p.

    See also Pain stiff.

STIFFNESS: *Acon.*, Agaric., *Bell.*, *Bry.*, Calc., *Chel.*,
        Coccul., Col., *Dulc.*, *Ferr.p.*, Graph., *Ign.*,
        Kali c., Lach., Lachn., Nit. ac., Nux,
        *Phos.*, Phyt., *Rhus*, Sang., *Sulf.*, Zinc.

    L. side: *Acon.*, *Ferr.p.*, *Rhus.*

    R. side: *Acon.*, *Bell.*, *Bry.*, Col., Kali c., Phyt., *Sul.*

    And bruised feeling in l. side, extending to l.
        shoulder and back, <motion, > lying: Acon.

      Boring in nape: Psor.

      Contraction, with rheumatic pain in muscles of
          N. and back: China, Cim., Clem., Dulc.

      Heaviness of nape as from a heavy load, with pain-
          ful tension: Vinca m.

      Pain in upper cervical and dorsal muscles: Zinc.

      Paralyzed sensation in all limbs and N. during and
          after walking: Rhus.

      Rigidity from overstrain from lifting: Calc.

    From cold: Acon., Bell., Bry., Calc.p., Dulc., Ferr.p.

      Getting hair cut: Bell., Bry.,

STIFFNESS, from getting Head wet: Bell., Bry., Calc.
Cold air: Dulc.
Heaviness and weariness as from a load: Vinca m.
In side of N.: Dig.
N. head kept almost motionless: Plumb.
Dull, with rheumatic pain from slightest draught of air: Calc. p.
On moving head, with painfulness on deep breathing: Chel.
Painful: Merc.. Mez., Natr.
And tension: Colch., Dig.
Rheumatic: Calc., *Rhus*, Verat.
Sensation of, in l. side and nape, extending into ear: Thuya.
With tracking in vertebrae on moving N.: Chel:
With heaviness: Ginseng.
Neuralgia, < early A. M., and after eating or from touch: Nux.
STRETCHING of neck involuntarily: Lyc.
TEARING and jerking in: Lyc.
Drawing in: Clem.
In cords: Berb.
Muscles: Carbo v.
R. side: Iod., Zinc.
Side of, alt. with same in chest: Amm. m.
See also Pain tearing.
TENDER, N., to touch with pain: Kalm.
TENDERNESS and much swelling if N.: Ail.
TENSION and heaviness of muscles of nape: Chel.
Stiffness: Carbo an.
In muscles: Carbo an., Cic., Chel., Lyc.
THICKENING, apparent, of N.: Con.
THIGHS, bruised sensation in hips and N. and: Phos. ac.
TIGHTENING around: Glon.
TIRED, feels: Fagrop.
TOO WEAK to support head: Calc. p., Natr. m.
It falls from side to side: Calc. p.
TREMBLE, N. and head shake and: Carbo v.
TUMORS, fatty, of N. and back: Bar. c.
VERTEBRAE, cracking in, with stiffness on moving N.: Chel.

VERTEX, violent pain in N. extending back and forth to
V.: Chel.

WALKING, sensation of a load on neck, and paralyzed
feeling in feet during and after: Rhus.

WEAKNESS of cervical and dorsal muscles, with heaviness of head: Caps., Coccul., Plat., Verat.

WEARINESS and lameness in: Aesc.

Of feet, with rheumatic pain in nape: Puls.

WEARY, muscles of, grow: Glon.

WEIGHT, feeling of: Phos.

WRITING, tensive pain in nape and occiput while: Lyc.

Weariness in N. evenings while: Zinc.

---

# SHOULDERS AND ARMS.

ACHES and pains in S.: Calc. p.

ACHING and tenderness on top of r. trapezius: Phyt.

In both S. when at rest, with bruised pain: Lyc.

< l., pain from head to S.: Hydrast.

S.: Apis.

Bruised: Hydrast., Lyc.

Moves from teeth to A.: Mang. ox.

R. S. and A., A. feels as if bruised, at times cannot
raise A.: Nit. ac.

ALIVE, sensation of something, in S. joint: Berb.

AXILLA, itching in: Staph.

Sticking beneath r.: Sulf.

See also Glands.

BEATEN; A. painful even at rest as if humerus were: Puls.

See also Neuralgia and Pain beaten.

BLOW, painful strokes as from a heavy, on middle of l.A.:
Anac.

BORING and drawing in S. joint: Col.

In A.: Cina, Plumb. ac., Zinc.

Anterior part of A., with lacerating in teeth:
Plumb. ac.

L. S.: Aur. met.

R. S. from biceps to elbow: Ferrum.

Tearing in l. S. joint: Rhod.

BOTH A. painfully difficult to move: Thuya.

Fixed in pronate position: Plumb.

BROKEN and dislocated feeling in A.: Puls.

BRUISED, A.: Arn., Bapt., Bufo, Clem., Led., Natr. m.,
Nit. ac.

And sore feeling in S.: Con.

Deltoid feels as if, when touched: Acon.

Feeling in A.: Arn., Clem., Cic.

~L. S.: Kali i.

Violent stitches in S. as if: Iod.

See also Aching and Pain bruised.

BURNING throbbing in A.: Bell.

See also Deltoid.

CAN move A. laterally but cannot raise them: Sang.

COLD, A. feel, when raising them: Verat.

COLDNESS and insensibility of A.: Acon.

In A. which no amount of clothing can remove: Sang.

CONSTRICTED: See Pain cramplike.

CORNERS: See Pain in.

CRACKING, audible, of l. S. joint, on every motion: Bar. c.

CRACKING in S. joint on bending A. backward and inability to raise A. on account of pain as
if dislocated: Thuya.

Of S. joints: Ferrum.

See also Creaking.

CRAMPS of A.: Cup.

CRAMPY drawing in region of r. biceps when writing: Val.

Jerking through humerus: Val.

Tearing in A.: Bell., Val.

Darting like an electric shock, repeated through
humerus, intensely painful: Val.

See also Pain crampy or cramplike.

CRAWLING sensation in A.: Sec.

Tearing in A.: Cham.

CREAKING in r. S. joint, with bruised pain on touch,
shooting and tearing through A., inability to raise A.: *Ferrum.*

CUTTING drawing across S. above deltoid: Spig.

See also Jerks.

DARTING tearing in A.: Carbo v., Val.

See also Pain darting.

DELTOID, burning painful spot in, with external heat:
Nux.

Jerking in: Sulf.

More r.: Kalm.

DELTOID, Pinching in l.: Fluo. ac.

R.: Ferrum.

Pressure at insertion of r.: Hyperic.

Quivering jerks in muscles: Ign.

Swollen, feels as if bruised when touched: Acon.

Twitching in: Ign.

See also Digging and Pain at.

DIGGING pinching in r. deltoid on raising A.: Bufo.

DISLOCATED and broken feeling in A.: Puls.

Sprained feeling in l. S., > violent motion: Niccol.

See also Pain dislocated.

DRAWING and boring in S. joint: Col.

Paralytic stiffness of A.: Acon.

Tearing in S.: Col.

From below axilla to middle of A. on raising A.: Rhus.

Goutlike in S.: Canst.

In A.: Acon., Agaric., Bell., Lyc., Puls., Rhus, Sulf.

Humeri after midnight: Sulf.

Stiffness in muscles of l. A.: Verat.

Stitches in A., from S. down: Rhus.

Tearing in A.: Carbo an., Rhus, Sulf.

FALLING inert of A. when lifted: Con.

FATIGUED, A. easily, from moderate exercise, so that everything held is allowed to fall: Stann.

And powerless; A. are: Sep.

FEMUR, dislocated feeling in, when sitting: Ipec.

FINGERS jerking and stitches in A. and: Cic.

Numbness from S. to tips of: Ox. ac.

FOREHEAD, tearing or wandering in r. S., alt. with pain in: Bry.

GLANDS, painful swelling of axillary: Rhus.

GOUTLIKE drawing in S.: Canst.

GURGLING feeling in S.: Berb.

HANDS, paralytic lacerating along A. to: Sabin.

As if powerless: Acon.

Tied to body: Abrot.

HEADACHE extending over S.: Glon.

HEAVINESS and exhaustion of A. on motion: Carbo v.

Tiredness in S.: Carbo an., Ginseng.

Of A.: Bell., Carbo v., Canst., Gels., Led., Sil.

Paralytic, with weak A.: Nux.

HIP, rheumatism of l. S. and r.: Nux m.

HUMERUS, feeling of weight in: Sulf.

Heaviness with tension in: Sulf.

JERKING and sticking in A. and fingers: Cic

Stitches: Cic.

In A.: *Cic.*, Cup., Iod.

Muscles of A. when resting it: Stann.

Tearing, paralytic, on top of S. with sensitiveness to touch, pain renewed by touch even of coat: China.

JERKS, painful cutting, from r. S., toward head: Cham.

JOINTS, boring and drawing in, of S.: Col.

Cracking of S.: Thuya.

Cramp and stiffness in, of A.: Phos. ac.

Neuralgia of S., and A.: Staph.

Pressure, painful in A. near elbow: Sabin.

Sticking, extremely painful in S., on raising A.: Led.

Stiffened by Rheumatism: Fluo. ac.

See also Creaking and Pain.

LACERATING, paralytic, along A. to hands: Sabin.

See also Pain lacerating.

LOSS of power of a: Cham., Chel., Gels., Zinc.

NEURALGIA in brachial plexus as if bruised or beaten: Verat.

See also Joint.

NUMBNESS from S. to tips of fingers: Ox. ac.

In A.: Acon., Cim., Glon., Nux.

PAIN, about l. S. with cardiac troubles: Asparag.

Aching and soreness as if beaten: *Arn.*, *Eup. per.*, Sul.

In A.: Arn., Bell., Eup. per., Mang. ox., Stram.. Sul.

S.: Apis.

Moves from teeth to A.: Mang. ox.

Across S.: Ars.

Acute rheumatic: Agar.

And aches in S.: Calc. p.

Arthritic tearing in r. S.: Sil.

Beaten, as if, in A.: *Arn.*, *Eup. per.*, Sul.

S.: Stram.

Blows, as from, under r. S. when moving or touching it.: Kali c.

PAIN, Boring in S.: Mez., Nitrum.

Pinching in A.: Cina.

Breaking in A.: Calc.p.

Bruised aching in S.: Hydrast., Lyc.

In both, $<$ l.: Hydrast.

And crushing in A.: Bufo.

As if in A.: *Arn.*, *Led.*, Natr.m.

S.: Dros., Natr., Nux.

In A.: *Arn.*, Bufo, *Led.*, Natr. m., Nit. ac.

Bone of A.: Hep.

Muscles of r. S.: Led.

S.: Ferr., Hydrast., Led., Lyc., Thuya.

And between S. as after a heavy load, even the clothing is oppressive: Granat.

On touch, shooting and tearing through upper A. cannot raise A.: Ferrum.

Or sprained, as if, in l. S.: Sulf.

Contractive, tensive, in deltoid when laying hand on table: Asarum.

Constant in S. joints: Puls.

Cramplike, close to S., as if in chest, as if everything were tightly constricted: Plat.

In A.: Calc. p., Col.

Crushing and bruised: Bufo.

Dislocated, as if in A.: Coccul., Mag. c.

Joints of S., if he raises A. high or puts them under head while in bed: Oleand.

S.: Caps., Ign., Mag. c.

From, in S. on motion: Mag. c.

Joint, after exertion: Sep.

Deltoid, at r., just above insertion of biceps, causing inability to move A. or fingers: Ferrum.

Drawing, beginning at S.: Apis.

From S. to wrist, in transient recurring attacks: Puls.

Fingers: Nux.

Drawing from small of back to S.: Ars.

In A.: Agar., Bell., Lyc., *Puls.*, *Rhus.*,*Sulf.*

Inner side of l. A., weakness of whole A.: Bell.

Surface of both: Lyc.

Joint and A.: Sulf.

L. S. and neck: Lill. t.

PAIN; Drawing in S.: Acon., Apis, Hep., Puls., Sulf.,
    See also Tearing.
    When lying on S. at night: Carbo v.
    Shooting in A.: Acon.
  Dull in A.: Fagop.
      S.: Aesc., Dios.
    Rheumatic in S.: Acon., Fagop.
    Sticking: Staph.
  During rest in S.: Colch., Rhus.
  Darting, crampy, like electric shocks repeatedly
      through humerus: Val.
  Extending inward, in A., near elbow: Sabin.
  Even at rest, as if, humerus were beaten: Puls.
  Flying in r. S.: Hyperic.
  From head to S.; aching in both, <1.: Hydrast.
    Fatigue: Natr. m.
    Liver to S. and hips: Viper. t.
  In A., even at rest, as if beaten: Puls.
    Bones of A.: Bufo, *Hep.*, Psor.
    Both S.: Kreos., *Lyc.*, Verat.
    A., cannot bear slightest motion: Cham.
    Deltoid muscle on raising A.: Bar. c.
    Forehead alt. with tearing or wandering in r. S.
      joint: Bry.
  Joints of A.: Cup.
      As if S. were dislocated: Caps., Ign.
      Of S. as if it would be torn asunder: Mez.
      S. on bending A. backward: CALC., *Ign.*,
          RHUS.
        As after violent exertion
        or as if bruised: Ign.
  L. S., Dios., Kalm., Spig.
    And A.: Kalm.
    Extending to heart: Magnol.
  R. deltoid, sore to touch, on a place size ˙of hand:
      Lob. i.
    S., and A., <writing: Merc. iod.
      Joint and head, can hardly raise A.: Mag. c.
        Near insertion of pectoralis major, at
          margin of muscle: Lith. c.
  Muscles of r. A.: Verat.
  S., A. and tips of fingers, whole flesh sore, no>
      from sweat (Merc.): Chel.

PAIN; Just below joint so that he could not raise A. high or put it across back: CALC.

Lacerating in A.: Plumb., Sabin.

S. and joint, <nights: Sulf.

Teeth with boring in interior part of A.: Plum. ac.

Lame in A. and thighs: Coccul.

Lameness or stitches, as from, in r. S.: Lauro.

Like a pressing down in S.: Merc.

L. S., in: Ambra. Bell., Dios., *Ferr.*, Graph., Hydrast., *Kalm.*, Kali c., *Phos.*, RHUS, *Spig.*, *Staph.*

Of l. S. with rheumatism: Ferr. Kalm., Spig., *Sulf.*

On top of l. S. Rhus.

R. S.: Sang.

Near point of r. pectoralis major, at margin of muscle: Lith. c.

Paralytic in A.: Clem., *Colch.*, Dulc., *Staph.*

Jerking, on top of S., which is painfully sensitive to touch: China.

Pressive in l. A. <touch and motion: Staph.

Pressed against sharp corners, as if S. were: Kreos.

Pressive in S.: Lauro., Nit. ac., Nitrum, Staph.

Bones of S.: Lauro., Nit. ac., Nitrum.

On S.: Nit. ac.

Violent, in l. S., no>from motion: Staph.

Rheumatic esp. in l. S.: Sulf.

In A.: *Calc.p.*, *Sulf.*

Near S. joint, cannot raise A.: Calc.p.

Both S.: Berb., CALC., *Bry.*, Hydrast., Ign., Iris, Lyc., Nux, Rhod., Puls., RHUS, SULF.

<nights: Kali bi.

Elbow, forearm, r. S. and first finger of l. hand: Hydrast.

L. S.: Rhus, *Sulf.*

And A., in region of deltoid, <raising A. upward and and backward: RHUS.

R. S., elbow, forearm and first finger of l. hand: Hydrast.

Joint, goes to upper A. and elbow joint: Lob. i.

Region of l. deltoid and A.; Rhus.

On top of S.: Bry.

PAIN; Rheumatic, paralytic in r. S.: Puls., Rhod.

With stitches over l.
eye: Berb.

Paralytic in r. S. mornings when resting upon
it, sometimes extends below elbow:
Rhod.

Raging in A.: Thuya.

Pinching in r. deltoid: FERRUM.

Rheumatic near S. joint, cannot raise A.: Calc. p.

R. S., in: Berb., *Bry.*, FERR. Hydrast., Iris, Lith.
c., *Mag.*, *Mez.*, *Phyt.*, Puls., Rhod., *Sang.*

S. in both: Alum., Ambra, CALC., Caps., Chel.,
China, Dios., FERR., Graph., Hydrast.,
*Ign.*, Iris, Led., Lith. c., Lyc., *Mag.c.*
Merc., *Mez.*, Nit. ac., Nux. $_m$. and v.,
*Phos.*, Puls., RHUS, *Sang.*, *Staph.*, *Sulf.*,
Thuya.

Severe. in S.: Acon., Fagop., Ferr., Puls., Sep.

Both S. joints: Puls.

L. S. joint: Fagop.

S. joint as if it would drop off: Acon.

Be torn off: Sep.

Sharp, tensive, in r., <motion, esp. raising A.: Iris

Shooting in A.: Form.

S.: Form.

R. S. joint with stiffness and inability to
raise A.: Phyt.

Through A.: Calc., Ferr., *Rhus.*

Sprain, as from a. in A.: Euphorb.

Sprained, in l. S. joint on motion, twisting or raising
A.: Vespa c.

R. S. on motion: Staph.

Joint: Sabina.

A. when carrying it upward and backward: Calc., RHUS.

S. joints, drawing and turning A. up,
returns on letting A. hang down
or lie on anything: Ruta.

Sticking, extremely painful in S. joint on motion or
raising A.: Led.

Tensive, in r. S., <motion esp. raising A.: *Iris.*

Stitching, as if beaten in A. (r.): Verat.

Darting, in A.: Form.

Swollen and sore, as if, in S.: Cup.

PAIN; Tearing and drawing, in and between S., prevents
sleep: Bor.
Constant, in S. joints: Puls.
In l. S. joint, with a sprained paralyzed
feeling: Ambra:
S.: Ambra, Puls.
Torn asunder, as if S. would be: Mez.

Twitching, violent, from l. S. joint to middle finger:
Arn.
Weight, as of in: S. Hep.

PAINFUL, A. even at rest as if humerus were beaten:
Puls.
Numbness of A.: Cim.

Pressure in A. near elbow joint: Sabin.

Strokes as from a heavy blow on middle of A.: Anac.

Weakness of A.: Cic.

Weariness of A.: Bufo, Calc.

PARALYZED, l. S. seems: Rhus.

PARALYSIS of A.: Cup., Sulf.

With tearing on r. A.: Sulf.

PARALYTIC jerking, tearing on top of S.: China.

Lacerating along A. to hands: Sabin.

Pressure in A.: Bell., Cyc.

Sensation in A.: Cina, *Rhus*.

Stiffness and drawing in A.: Acon.

Tearing and jerking in A.: Cham.

Weakness in A.: Bufo, Dig., Gels., *Stann.*

If a light weight is held even for a
short time: Stann.

PRESSURE and tension, painful, of r. S. at rest: Bry.

In A.: Hell., *Kalm.*, Sabin.

Above l. elbow, prevents putting on coat alone:
L. A.: Kalm.                     [Colch.

Muscles of A.: Hell., Kalm.

R. axilla, <touch: Agnus.

S. or in joint: Lauro.
On S.: Canst.

Top of r. S., >touch, becoming a sticking on
deep breathing, which extends downward
and outward to S. joint: Bry.

Painful in A. near elbow joint: Sabin.

L. S. or both joints: Led.
Shooting or stitching on top of l. S. Bell.

PULSATING stinging in r. S. joint: Osmium.

QUIVERING in r. S., at rest: Dros.

RAISE, inability to, A.: Calc., FERR., Mag.c., Rhus, Sang.

Upward and backward: Calc., Rhus.

RHEUMATIC drawing in S.: Bry., Carbo v., Puls., Sulf.

Tension in S.: Lyc.

RHEUMATISM and pain of l. S.: Ferr., Kalm., SULF.

Muscular of S.: Amm. canst.

Of A.: Bell., Carbo an., *Calc.p.*, Kalm., Lyc., Mang. ox., Rhus, Stann., Sulf., Val.

L. A.: Anac., Bell., *Calc.*, *Kalm.*, Magnol., Mang. ox., *Rhus*, Staph., Zinc.

S.: *Ferr.*, *Kalm.*, Nux, *Rhus*, SULF.

Andr. hip: Nux m.

R. A.: Bell., Carbo an., Graph., *Ferr.*, *Sang.*,*Sulf.*

S.: Bell., *Bry.*, FERR., Calc., *Mag.c.*, Phyt., *Sang.*

And A „<night in bed: Ferr., Mag.e., Sang.

S.: *Bry.*, CALC., FERR., Ign., Iris, Kalm.,*Mag.*,˙ Nux, Nux m., RHUS, Phyt., SANG., SULF.

And hip: Carbol. ac.

Knee: Kreos.

Hip and knee (l.): Verat. v.

And knee, r. side: Apoc. and.

Trapezius: Sang.

Pain extends to upper part of chest,<motion: Ferr. p.

So that A. could not be raised: Kalm.

<nights, hands and fingers feel swollen: Nitrum.

RIGID, A. nearly: Ferr.

SHOCK, crampy, darting, tearing like an electric: Val.

SHOOTING and tearing in A.: Form.

SHUDDERING or thrilling in region of l. S.: Verat. v.

SINK down exhausted, A.: Lach.

SLEEP, A. go to: Carbo v., Cham., Coccul.

SORE, S. painfully, to touch, also A.: Ferr.

Tender and swollen, A.: Graph.

SORENESS and aching in A.: *Eup. perf.*

Stiff feeling about S., and chest: Bapt.

SPRAINED, paralyzed feeling, with tearing in l. S.: Ambra.

STICKING and jerking in A. and fingers: Cic.

 Extremely painful, in S. joint on raising A.: Led.

 In A.: Cann. s., Coccul., Dros.

  S.: Graph., *Iris*, Led., Thuya.

   Joint and A., during rest: Coccul.

    <touch and motion: Staph.

 Lightninglike in r. S.: Papaya v.

 On motion, extending from S. to chest: Sulf.

 So that A. could not be raised without crying aloud: Cic.

 Violent, also tearing in l. S.: Graph.

STIFFNESS, of S , mornings on washing, with pressure in S. and heaviness of A.: Phos.

STINGING in A.: Sabin.

  R. S., during motion, <raising A., with tension: Iris.

STITCH in r. axilla, extending into chest: Sulf.

 Severe on raising A.: Led.

STITCHES, drawing from S. down through A.: Rhus.

 In A.: Cham., Dros., Rhus, Sulf.

  S. joints and A. at rest: Coccul.

   On raising A.: Sulf. ac.

 Inward in l. S. with throbbing: Rhus.

 On top of S. at every inspiration: Hyperic.

 Sharp, on top of r. S.: Guiac.

 Violent, in S. as if bruised: Iod.

 When lying, in S., >moving: Rhus.

STITCHING pressure on top of l. S.: Bell.

STRETCHING and twisting in A.: Bell.

SWOLLEN, A.: *Crotal. h.*

  R.: Graph.

 Sore and tender, A.: Graph.

 S., deltoid feels as if bruised when touched: Acon.

TEARING and burning in S., A. lame: Rhus.

 In A.: Carbo an., Indigo, Lauro., Rhus, Sulf., Zinc.

  L. A.: Zinc.

   S.: Stann.

    Esp. at night in bed: Phos.

    With a sprained paralyzed feeling: Ambra.

  R. A., with paralysis: Sulf.

   Severe when raising it: Carbo an.

  S., as if it would be torn asunder: Mez.

   Joint, <motion: Led.

TEARING in S.: Ambra, Bry., Kali c., Lyc., Mez., Phos., Puls., Stann., Zinc.

Joint and on top of scapula: Rhus.

Obliging one to bend A.: Puls.

Near l. S.: Zinc.

Paralytic, along r. A. to hand: Sabin.

Pressure in A.: Bell., Led.

Top of l. S.: Cann. s.

See also Pain tearing.

TENSION and drawing in S.: Pet.

Tearing in both S.: Zinc.

In l. A. in open air: Rhus.

Pectoral and dorsal muscles at S. joint, <raising A.: Hyos.

R. S. during rest with pressure: Bry.

Painful, in r. S. when at rest: Bry.

Rheumatic, in r. S. joint: Lyc.

THIGHS and S. very weary: Thuya.

THRILLING through A.: CANN. I.

THROBBING burning in A.: Bell.

Painful in r. S.: Led.

TREMBLING in A.: Bell., Calc. p., Cim.

TWISTING and stretching in A.: Bell.

In A.: Bell., Iod.

TWITCH, first in l., later in r. deltoid: Ox. ac.

TWITCHING about l. S. joint: Spong.

In r. S. during rest: Dros.

Of muscles of l. S.: Spong.

VERY lame in A.: Iris, Rhus.

WEAKNESS in A. (great) : Phos.

Of l. A., difficulty in moving or raising it: *Calc.*, Ferr.

Paralytic, in A. if light weight is held for a short time: Stann.

WEARINESS in A.: Glon., Hep.

In S.: Lauro., Thuya.

WEIGHT on S., esp. l. near clavicle: Rhus.

When walking in open air: Sulf.

Violent pain in S. joints on lifting the lightest: Sep.

## UPPER EXTREMITIES.

ACHING: Carbol. ac., Eup. perf.

> As if bruised above and below elbow, with soreness: Eup.

> In l. and r. wrist: Carbol. ac.

ARM, aching in l. and r. wrist: Carbol. ac.

ASLEEP, falling, of the one on which he rests his head, during sleep: Rhus.

> On awaking mornings: Calad.

> With crawling sensation: Coccul.

AWAKING, asleep on: Calad.

BODY, feel as if tied to: Abrot.

BONES, paralytic tearing in, jerking, <touch: China.

BURSTING feeling in, on letting them hang down: Viper. t.

CARRIAGE, feel as if gone to sleep when riding in a: Form.

COLDNESS in, which no amount covering can>: Sang.

CRAMP in r. drawing it backward: Amm. c.

CRAWLING sensation: Coccul.

DRAWING in: Nit. ac., Rhus.

> L. at night, with paralyzed sensation: *Rhus*.

ELBOW: See pain aching.

FINGERS, numbness from shoulder to tips: Ox. ac.

> Tearing stitches along r. to tips: Caps.

GANGRENE: Ars., Carbo v., Ran. flam., Sil.

> And inflammation: Ran. flam.

HANDS, leaden heaviness with difficulty of using muscles of wrists and: Curare.

> See also Pain paralytic.

HEAD, sensation as if H. and U. E. were too large: Aranea, Bapt.

HEAVINESS: Curare, Bell., Natr. m.

> And paralytic feeling: Bell.

> Leaden, difficulty in using muscles, <wrists and hands: Curare.

> Weakness and sinking down: Natr. m.

INFLAMMATION and gangrene: Ran. flam.

JERKING in: Cup.

 Involuntary, of arms and fingers: Cic.

 Tearing, paralytic, in bones, $<$touch: China.

LAMENESS and pressure with weakness: Bell.

NEURALGIA and numbness from suddenly checked perspiration: Acon., Acon. unct.

NUMB, become while at work: Phos.

NUMBNESS: Acon., Acon. unct., Curare, Nux, Ox. ac.,
 And tingling of l.: Acon.        Phos.

 From shoulders to tip of fingers: Ox. ac.

 See also Neuralgia.

PAIN; Arn., Bapt., Calc., Carbol. ac., Eup. perf., Colch.,
    Rhus, Scroful.

 Aching: Carbol. ac., Eup. perf.

  As if bruised, above and below elbow, with
    -  soreness: Eup. perf.

 In l. arm and r. wrist: Carbol. ac.

 And swelling: Rhus.

 Bruised, as if: Arn., Bapt., Calc., Eup. perf.

    On moving or taking hold of U.E.: Calc.

  With dingy red marbled spots: Berb.

 Buzzing: Scroful.

 In joints when bending them back: Ign.

 On motion, as if humerus were lying loosely in joint
    and would be easily dislocated: Croc.

 Paralytic in all joints on motion: ARN., Calc.

    So that the slightest thing cannot be held
      in the hands on account of the
      violency of the: Colch.

 Rheumatic, in elbow, r. shoulder, forearm and first
    finger of l. hand: Hydrast.

  L., from shoulder or elbow to wrist:
          Guiac.

 Shooting: Rhus.

 Tearing, violent, $<$lying still: Rhus.

PAINFULNESS and swelling: Rhus.

PARALYZED, hang as if: Acon.

 Sensation in l.: Plat.

PARALYSIS begins in, and travels downward (Led.,
        reverse.) Merc.

 Rheumatic, $<$r.: Canst.

PARALYTIC feeling and heaviness: Bell.

 Hard pressure as though deep in muscles or periosteum: Cyc.

PARALŸTIC jerking tearing in bones, <touch: China.

    See also Pain paralytic.

PRESSURE and lameness with weakness: Bell.

    Hard deep, as if in periosteum: Cyc.

RHEUMATIC paralysis, <l.: Rhus.
                    <r.: Canst.

RHEUMATISM: Caust., Chel., Colch ,. Ferr., Hydrast.,
           Kalm., Lyc., Puls., Rhus, Sang., Sulf.

    L. side: Kalm., Magnol., Rhus.

    R. side: Caps., Hydrast., Ferr., Sang.

SENSATION as if U. E. and head were too large: Aran.,
                            Bapt.

    Of stretching and twisting: Bell.

SHOOTING through, extends in l. and out of finger tips,
                    with drawing: Rhus.

    See also Pain shooting.

SHOULDER, numbness from, to finger tips: Ox. ac.

SINKING down feeling with heaviness : Natr. m.

SLEEP, feeling as if gone to, when riding in a carriage:
                          Form.

    Go to, immediately on grasping anything firmly:
                        Cham.

SPOTS, dingy, red marbled, with bruised pain: Berb.

STIFFNESS and cramp in joints: Phos. ac.

STITCHING, tearing, along r. to finger tips: Caps.

STRETCHING and twisting, sensation of: Bell.

SWELLING and Painfulness: Rhus.

TEARING in r., with paralysis: SULF.

    Stitching along r. to finger tips: Caps.

    <lying still: Rhus.

    See also Pain tearing.

TIED to body, feel as if: Abrot.

TINGLING and numbness (Nux), of l.: Acon.

TOO large, sensation as if head and U. E. were: Aran.,
                          Bapt.

TREMBLING after moderate exertion: Rhus.

TWISTING and stretching, sensation of: Bell.

UNSTEADINESS of muscles: Caust.

WEAKNESS: Curare, Natr. m., Bell.

    And loss of power: Kali c.

    Heaviness and sinking down feeling: Natr. m.

    Of, as after long continued sickness, numbness as if
        a heavy weight hung to extremities, soreness of
        muscles, <attempting to lift anything: Curare.

WEAKNESS of R. arm and wrist, cannot raise anything:
Sil.
With lameness and pressure: Bell.
WEARINESS and lassitude: Arg. n.
WEIGHT, numbness as if a heavy, hung to U.E.: Curare.
WORK, become numb while at: Phos.

---

# ELBOWS.

ACHING and lameness on outer and under side of l. (above):
Abrot.
See also Pain aching.
ARM feels as if broken at r. joint, with a troublesome paralytic pain: Bry.
BORING in: Phos.
And pressure: Clem.
BROKEN, arm feels as if at r. joint: Bry.
BRUISED sensation: Led., Thuya, Val.
See also Pain bruised.
BURNING: Merc.
CRACKING in, joint: Merc.
CUTTING in: Bell.
DRAWING: Bry., Kali c., Natr. m., Nitrum, Zinc.
And tearing: Kali c., Zinc.
Cutting: Phos. ac.
Sticking: Carbo an.
Tearing: Acon., Canst.
See also Pain drawing.
FEEL as if broken: Bry.
GOUTLIKE drawing: CAUST., Guiac.
JERKING tearing in: RHUS.
JOINT, arm feels as if broken at r.: Bry.
Bubbling sensation in: Rheum.
Jerking tearing in: RHUS.
Painful to touch: Dros.
Swelling of r.: Bry.
KNEE, drawing in l. alt. with same in E.: Bry.
LAMENESS and aching on outer and under side of l., just
above E.: Abrot.

PAIN: Abrot., Aloe. Ars., Bufo, Bry., Carbo v., Plat.
    Aching, dull: Aesc.                  Puls.
    Bruised and weary: Natr. s.
           As if (in joint) : Carbo v.
           Extending from: Cyc.
    Contractive, pressive: Nux.
    Cutting: Bell.
    Drawing: Canst., Natr. c.
        In bone: China.
        Tearing: Acon., Canst.
    Dull aching: Aesc.
      Rheumatic: Acon.
    Gnawing, rheumatic: Indigo.
    Grinding: Dios.
    In bend: Graph.
      R.: Plat.
      Tendons, tensive, in bend of E. on moving arm:
    Paralytic, drawing: Bell., Cham.      Puls.
    Periodic: Kreos.
    Pressive, contractive: Nux.
    Rheumatic: Chel., Clem., Form., Kali bi., Lac. can.
        Extends from shoulder to E.: Chel.,Clem.
        Dull, about: Acon.
    Severe: Fagop.
    Shooting, extending through: Form.
    Sticking: Berb.
    Tearing, drawing: Acon., Canst.
    Tensive, in tendons on moving arm: Puls.
    Violent, in both: Hep.
    Weary and bruised: Natr. s.
PAINFULNESS of joints to touch: Dros.
PRESSING and boring: Clem.
PRESSURE: Dig.
SHOOTINGS through: Calc. p.
STICKING in outer condyles: Sabin.
STITCHES with swelling of r. joint: Bry.
SWELLING: Bry.
TEARING: Agaric., Kali c.. Lyc., Mez., Zinc.
TENSION as if too short: Sep.
ULNA, drawing in alt. with same in l. knee: Bry.
WRIST, jerking and tearing in, joint and W. during rest:
    *Rhus.*

# FOREARMS.

ACHING and soreness: Eup. perf.

COLDNESS, icy, of F. or only hands: Apis, Brom., Colch.

CRAMPS: Merc.

DRAWING: *Hep.*, *Oleand.*, *Sulf.*

    In r.: Oleand.

    Painful in flexor tendons of l.: Hep.

    Pressure with weakness: Bell.

    Slow, painful, as if in nerves, extending from elbows to wrists: Sulf.

    Tearing in extensors of l.: Hep.

    See also Pains drawing.

ELBOWS: See Drawing slow.

FINGERS, stiffness and loss of power of, and F., on motion: RHUS.

HANDS, icy coldness of F. or only: Apis, BROM., Colch.

    R. F. and, seem to be of immense size: Cup.

    Unsteadiness of muscles of F. and: Canst.

ICY coldness of F. or only hands: Apis, BROM., Colch.

JERKING tearing in ulna: Cup.

LOSS of power: RHUS.

NERVES: See Drawing slow.

NUMBNESS: Aranea, Opi.

    Of parts supplied by ulna nerve: Aranea.

PAIN; Acute rheumatic in L.: Acon.

    Beaten, as if: Arn., Eup. perf., *Natr.m.*, *Rhus.*

        In l.: *Rhus.*

    Bone, drawing in: China, Nitr. ac.

        In middle of long: Phyt.

        Were pressed, as if, in middle of l.: Verat. a.

    Breaking: Calc.p.

    Broken, as if something were: Cup.

    Bruised, violent: Cyc.

    Cramplike, in muscles: Calc., Cina, Col., Cup.

        In l.: Acon.

PAIN; Crampy: Calc., Cina, COL.

    Dislocated, as if, in radius: Coccul.

    Drawing bone: China, Nit. ac.

        In: China, Nit. ac., Sil., Staph., SULF.

        Tearing: Acon., Carbo v.

    Excruciating: Plumb.

    In, ending in wrist joint: Aloe.

        Middle of l.: Verat. a.

            Long bones: Phyt.

        Near middle: Dios.

        R. as if sprained: Natr.c.

        Radius, <motion or touch: Sabin.

    Paralytic: Cham.

    Rheumatic: Acon., Form., Indigo.

        Acute in l.: Acon.

        In r.: Form.

    Shooting: Form.

    Sprained, as if in r.: Natr. c.

    Violent, bruised: Cyc.

PAINFUL drawing in flexor tendons of l.: Hep.

        Slow, as if in nerves: *Sulf.*

PARALYTIC drawing pressure, with weakness in r., and arm: Bell.

    Pressure: Cyc.

    Sensation: Chel.

    See also Pain paralytic.

PRESSURE, paralytic: Bell., Cyc.

        Drawing, with weakness: Bell.

SIZE, r. hand and F. seem to be of immense: Aranea, *Cup.*

SORENESS and aching: Eup. perf.

STIFFNESS: *Rhus.*

    And loss of power of F. and fingers, on motion: *Rhus.*

SWELLING rapidly increases, F. twice its natural size: *Rhus.*

SWOLLEN: *Crotal.*, Rhus.

TEARING: Carbo v., Hep., Kali c., Nitr. ac., Phos.

    Drawing in extensors of l.: Hep.

    In upper portions: Kali c.

        Outer surface: Oleum. an.

    Jerking in ulna: Cup.

TWITCHING above l. wrist during rest: Spig.

    In muscles of l.: Tarax.

ULNA, drawing in, alt. with in l. knee: Bry.
UNSTEADINESS of muscles of F. and hand: Canst.
VIOLENT stitches through: Dros.
WEAK and trembling: Cim.
WRISTS: See Drawing, slow.

---

# WRISTS.

ANKLES, gout of W. and: Abrot.
    Lameness of W. and, after sprains: Ruta.
    Rheumatism of W. and, with puffy swellings: Ruta.
    See also Pain agonizing.
ARMS: See Pain aching.
BORING and drawing: Mez.
    In condyles: Carbo an.
BROKEN: See Pain broken.
BURSA: BENN. AC., RUTA.
CRACKING: Arn., Bufo, Merc.
    Slight and sensation of dislocation: Arn., Bufo.
                     In r.: Arn.
    Sticking and powerlessness: Merc.
DISLOCATED or sprained, feels as if: Ox. ac.
    See also Pain dislocated.
DISLOCATION of bones of W. and tarsus: Ruta.
         R., sensation: Arn.
DRAWING and boring: Mez.
         Tearing: Acon.
    Cutting: Phos. ac.
    See also Pain drawing.
DROP: PLUMB.
DULL tearing: Carbo v.
ELBOW, stitches dart from W. to, when bending fingers:
                            Acon.
FEET, rheumatism of r. W. and both: RUTA, Sticta.
FINGERS, stiffness of W. and, with pain: Caul.
    Stitches from W. to elbow, on closing: Acon.
    See also Pain.

GANGLIA on flexors: Ruta.
GREAT weakness: Mez.
GOUT of W. and ankles: Abrot.
HANDS: See Pain in.
JERKING, tearing: *Rhus.*
LAMENESS, general, of W. and ankles,  after sprains:
                                        *Calc.*, RUTA.
PAIN; Aching in r. W. and l. arm: Carbol. ac.
    Agonizing in W., fingers, ankles and toes: Act. s.
    Broken, dislocated or sprained,  as if: *Eup. perf.*
    Bruised: Nit. ac.
            In bones of W. and backs of hands: Ruta.
    Cutting, on closing hands: Caul.
    Dislocated, as if: Bufo, *Eup. perf.*, Nit. ac., Ox.  ac.
                In r.: Calc.
                Or sprained: Calc., *Eup.perf.*, Ox.ac.
        See broken.
    Drawing: Acon., Caust., Cham., Mez., Phos. ac.
    Extending to, from shoulders: Chel.
    In forearm ending in W.: Aloe.
      R. W. in cold wet weather, >motion: RHUS, Ruta.
      W. and fingers alt. with same in  forehead: Bry.
            With stiffness of fingers  and  cutting  pain  on
                    closing hand: Caul.
    Laming and tearing, in joints: Bry.
    Pinching and drawing: Natr.m.
    Pressive: Calc.p., Natr.m.
    Rheumatic: *Act.s.*, *Caul.*, Cim., Led., Rhus, RUTA.
    Severe: Caul.
    Stiffness, like a: Puls.
    Sprained, as if: ARN., Carbo an., Calc., Ox. ac. p.,
                                Pet., *Sulf.*
            Or. wrenched, <motion: Bry.
        See dislocated.
    Tearing: Bry., Sulf., Thuya, Zinc.
            And laming: Bry.
    With stiffness of fingers and cutting pain  on  closing
                    hand: Caul.
    Wrenched or sprained, <motion: Bry.
PAINFULNESS and swelling: Tarent. H.
PERMANENTLY flexed: Caust., Guiac., *Merc.*
PRESSURE: Natr.c.

RHEUMATISM: Abrot., Act. s., Arn., Bry., Calc., Caul., Caust., Carbo v., Cim., Eup. perf., Led., Ox. ac., Rhus, RUTA, Stict., Viol. od.

Of ankles and W., with puffy swellings: Ruta.

L.: Rhus.

R.: Arn., Carbol. ac., Rhus, RUTA, Stict., Viol. od.

And both feet: Ruta, Sticta.

Esp. in females: Viol. od.

W. and finger joints: Caul.

Index finger: Lach.

SENSATION of dislocation and slight cracking in r.: Arn.

SHOOTING from elbow down to W.: Acon.

In joint: Acon.

SPRAIN, stitches like a, at carpo-radial articulation: Verbasc.

SPRAINED, feel as if: Arn.

Or dislocated: Ox. ac.

R.: Calc.

Sensation in upper surface of l. on bending it: Rhus.

SPRAINS, chronic: Calc. fluo.

General lameness of W. and ankles, after: RUTA.

STIFFNESS: *Calc.*, Merc., *Rhus*, SULF.

See Pain with.

STITCHES dart from W. to elbow on bending fingers: Acon.

SWELLING: Bufo, Ruta.

About joints of W., knee and index finger: Lach.

TEARING: Berb., Bry., Calc., *Carbo v.*

In r: <violent motion: Ruta.

TREMBLING of: Oleand., Plumb.

WRENCHED: See Pain wrenched.

# HANDS.

AGREEABLE thrilling through: CANN. I.

AIR, sweat while walking in open: Agar.

ASLEEP, fall at night: Sil.

    And insensible, seem: Coccul.

    Go to: Carbo v., Coccul., Form., Nux, Sil.

BEATING in: Natr. s.

BECOME rigid: Merc.

    Stiff easily: Thuya.

BED, cold H., feet and knees in: Phos.

BENT toward little finger: Sep.

BLOTCHES, hard elevated on: Rhus v.

BLUENESS: Apis, Kali brom.

    Of H. and nails; Chin. ars.

BORING in palms: Mez.

BRUISED and lame, feel as if: Kali bi.

BURNING: Agaric., Lyc., *Sulf.*

    And itching as if frostbitten: Agaric.

    Redness: Lyc.

CHAPPED: Graph., Petr., Hep., Suls.

CLENCHED: Stram.

CLOSE, inability to: Lach.

COLD: Ambr., Aloe, Apis, Chel., Coccul. Kali brom., Kreos., Phos., Rum., Sep., Sulf., Tab.

    And pulseless; Acon.

    Alternately: Coccul.

    Before vomiting: Verat.

    H. and feet: *Bell., Merc.,* Plumb., *Rhus.*

        And knees, in bed (Carbo v.): Phos.

        Body warm: Tab.

        Head warm: Bell.

        Preventing sleep: Rum.

    Icy: Ambra, Sep., Tab.

    Long lasting: Ambra.

One hot, the other: Chel., Lyc.

COLD; Sweat and blue nails: Nitr. ac., Nux.

On: Brom., Kali bi., Lill.t.

When coughing: Rum.

COLDNESS of, great: Verat.

CONTRACTION in flexors: Canst., *Cup.*, Iod.

Of: Cann. s., Caust., Merc., p. a.

And fingers: Merc. p. a.

COUGH, cold, with: Rum.

COULD not dress her child or herself, at times, without gloves, as it set her teeth on edge, as by strong acids: Tarent. C.

CRAMP: CUP., Dulc., Euphorb., Merc., SEC., Sil.

Of H. and feet: Cup., Euphorb.

So that nothing could be held: Cup., Euphorb.

CRAMPLIKE: See Lameness and Pain cramplike.

CRAWLING and fuzzy feeling in H. and feet: Hyperic.

Sensation: Hyperic., *Sec.*

DARKNESS and lividness of, and lower parts of fore-arms: Ars.

DEAD, feel when sewing: Crot.h.

DRAWING: *Nitr.ac.*, Oleum an.

Rheumatic, and sticking: Euphr.

See also Pain drawing.

DROPS things from weakness: Bov.

DRY, skin of palms and soles, very: Hep., Merc. p. a. Sulf.

DRYNESS, feeling of, in H. and fingers: Anac.

DULL itching in palms: Rann. bulb.

See Pain dull.

EATING, H. trembles while, the more it is raised the more it trembles: Coccul.

EMACIATION of, with lacerating pains: Sel.

FACE, sensation as if H., head and, were swollen: Aeth.

FEEL monstrously large: Aranea, Cann. i.

FEET and H. cold: Aloe, Phos., Sep., Tab.

Icy: Sep., Tab.

Body warm: Tab.

Preventing sleep: Aloe.

Cold H., feet and knees in bed: Phos.

Cramp of H. and: Cup., Euphorb.

See also Crawling. Rheumatism, Trembling.

FINGERS, H. bent towards little: Sep.

See also Contraction, Dryness, Stinging.

FOREARM and H. dark and livid: Ars.

R. seem to be of immense size: Aranea, Cann.i.

FROZEN, burning and itching in, as if: Agaric.

FUZZY and crawling feeling in H. and feet: Hyperic.

GLOVES: See Could.

HEAD, sensation as if H., face and, were swollen: Aeth.

HEAT of one, coldness of the other: Chel., Lyc.

Redness and swelling: Hep., Lact. ac.

With distended veins: Led.

HEAVINESS of: BELL.

HORNY spots on, like warts: Ant. c.

HOT swelling of joints: *Hep.*

ICY coldness, long lasting of: Ambra.

Of H. and feet: Sep., Tab.

Body warm: Tab.

INABILITY to close: Lach.

INSECTS, stinging in H. and fingers as from: Ambra.

INSENSIBLE and asleep, seem to be: Coccul.

Numb: Caust.

H. are: Acon., Ars., Canst., Coccul.

Palms are: Acon.

INVOLUNTARY shaking of: Lyc.

ITCHING and burning as if frozen: Agaric.

In palms: *Hep.*, *Ran. bulb.*, SULF.

Dull: Ran. bulb.

JERKING and twisting in: Iod.

In: Cup., Iod.

When holding pen: Stann.

JOINTS: See Hot and Pain dislocating.

KNEES, cold H., feet and, in bed: Phos.

Swelling of H. and legs to: Ferr.

Tendons in palms and under, contracted: Caust.

LAME, feel bruised and: Kali bi.

LAMENESS: Agar., Cann. s., Dios., Sil.

And cramplike pain, after slight exertion: Sil.

Cramplike: Cup., Sil.

Sudden: Cann. S.

LARGE, feel monstrously: Aranea, Cann. i.

LEGS, swelling of H., and to knees: Ferr.

LIVID, H. and lower parts of forearms dark and: Ars.

LOSS of power, cannot hold anything in H.: Hell.

NAILS, blueness of H. and: Chin. ars.

          With cold sweat on H.: *Nitr. ac.*, Nux̄.

NUMB: Acon., Bufo, Caust., Opi.

    And insensible: Canst.

        Stiff: Bufo.

        Tingling: Acon.

OEDEMA: Apis.

OSTEITIS of phalanges: Staph.

PAIN; Acute, sudden, in ball of r. thumb, extends up to r.

                shoulder: Ced.

    Beaten, as if: Bell., Dros.

        Or bruised, as if: Arn., Bapt., Bell., Dros.,

                Eup. perf.

    Bruised: See beaten.

    Cramplike, and lameness after slight exertion: Sil.

    Dislocating, in joints: Bell.

    Drawing: Arg. m., Arn., Canth., Cham., Merc., Puls.

        In ball of l. thumb alt. with same in occiput:

                Arg. m.

        Back: Staph.

        Violent, on ulna side of dorsum of r.: Arn.

    Dull, pressive: Kali c.

    In bones: Bell., Hep.

     Palms: Col.

     Phalanges, at night: Iris.

    Lacerating, with emaciation: Sel.

    Paralytic: Cham.

        Weakness, as from: Act. s.

    Pressive, dull: Kali c.

    Pricking: Glon.

    Rheumatic: Caul., Led., Phyt., Rhus.

    Stinging: Apis, Fagop.

    Sudden acute, in ball of r. thumb: Ced.

    Weakness, as from paralytic: Act. s.

PAINFUL sensation on palms and dorsal surface: Tarent. H.

PALMS, boring in: Mez.

        Itching in: *Hep.*, *Ran. bulb.*, SULF.

           Dull: Ran. bulb.

    See Painful, Knees.

    Warts on H., even P. covered: Anac.

PARALYTIC weakness, pain as from: Act. s.

    Weakness: Bufo, Crot. h.

    See Pain paralytic.

PARALYZED, flexor muscles: Gels.

PARALYSIS; and weariness: Cup.

PHALANGES, tearing in: Kali bi.
>   See Pain in.

POWERLESSNESS: Hell., Lyc.

PULSELESS and cold: Acon.

REDNESS and burning: Lyc.
>   Heat and swelling: Hep., Lac can.

RHEUMATIC drawing and sticking: Euphr.
>   Tearing in: Graph.
>   See also Pain rheumatic.

RHEUMATISM: Act. s., Ambr., Arn., Arg. n., CAUL.,
>>   Canst., Ferr., Graph., Hep., *Led.*,
>>   Merc., *Rhus*, Sel., Sil., Zinc.
>   Of backs, fingers swollen and bent: Amm p.
>>   L.: Oleand., *Rhus*.
>>   R.: Arn., Ced.

RIGID, become: Merc.

SENSATION as if H., head and face were swollen: Aeth.
>>   And arms were enormously enlarged
>>   (Cup., Cann. i.), each night, often
>>   strikes a light to see if it were
>>   really so; tremulous sensitiveness
>>   and exhaustion: Aranea.

SEWING, H. feel dead, when: Crot. h.

SHAKING involuntary: Lyc.

SHOULDER: See Pain sudden.

SHUT firmly: Phyt.

SIZE, H. seem of immense: Aranea, Cup.

SKIN: See Dry.

SLEEP prevented by cold feet and: Aloe.

SORE and stiff: Ferr.

SPOTS, horny on H. like warts: Ant. c.

STIFF and numb: Bufo.
>   Easily become: Thuya.
>   L. excessively: Oleand.

STINGING in H. and fingers as from insects: Ambra.
>   See also Pain stinging.

SUDDEN lameness: Cann. s.

SWEAT: Agar., Nit. ac., Nux.
>   Cold: Brom., Kali bi., Lill. t.
>>   With blue nails: Nit. ac., Nux.
>   While walking in open air: Agar.

SWELLING: Ferr., Hep., LAC CAN., Rhus.

    Great: Rhus.

    Heat and redness: Form., Hep.

    Hot, of joints: *Hep.*

    Of H. and legs to knees: Ferr.

    Rapidly: Phos.

SWOLLEN: See Sensation.

TEARING: Berb., Canst., Col., Zinc.

    In backs: Zinc.

        Joints: Col., Kali bi.

        Phalanges: Kali bi.

TENDONS in palms and under knees contracted: Canst.

THRILLING, agreeable, in: CANN. I.

TINGLING and numbness: Acon.

TREMBLING: *Agar.*, Caust., *Cim.*, China, Crot. h., Hep.,
           *Led.*, *Merc.*, *Phos.*, *Plumb.*, Zinc.

    And unsteadiness: Hep.

        Weakness: Cim., Zinc.

    Of, and feet: Merc.

        Could not write: Merc.

    On taking hold of, or moving them: Led.

    While eating, the higher the H. is raised the more it
                     T.: Coccul.

        Writing: China, Merc.

TREMOR: *Agar.*, Calc., Plumb.

TWITCHING and jerking: Iod.

UNSTEADINESS and Trembling: Hep.

VEINS distended with heat: Led.

    Swollen: Chel.

WALKING, H. sweat while, in open air: Agar.

WARTS: Anac., Ant. c., Natr. s., Thuya.

    H. and even palms covered: Anac.

    Horny spots on, like: Ant. c.

WEAKNESS: Act. s., Bov.. Cim., Zinc.

        And trembling: Cim., Zinc.

                While writing: Merc., Zinc.

    Drops things: Bov.

    Pain as from paralytic: Act. s.

WENS between metacarpal bones: Phos. ac.

WEARINESS and paralysis: Cup.

WRITING, H. tremble while: China, Zinc.

            And feet: Merc.

        And weak while: Zinc.

# FINGERS.

ACHING: Dios., Fagop., Thuya.

    And tiredness while writing: Fagop.

    In joints: Cann. s.

AIR, tips of, sensitive to cold: Cistus.

ANKLES: See Pain agonizing.

ARTHRITIC nodosities in, joints: Clem., Led.

                  Chronic: Amm. p., Ben. ac., Calc., Guiac., Staph.

ARTHRITIS rheumatoid: Calc.

BLACK: See Injured and Nails become.

BLUE nails from coldness: Nux. *Verat.*

BONES, sticking in of, little F.: Cann. s.

BORING in joints: Aur. met.

    See Pain boring.

BRITTLE, nails extremely: ALUM., *Sil.*, Thuya.

BURNING in: Berb., Fagop., *Zinc.*

      First joints and phalanges: Zinc.

      Joints, as if from needles: Berb.

CLENCHED, can not be: Caul., Dig.

COLD air, tips sensitive to: Cist.

    Joints become yellow and: Chel.

    Tips covered with, sweat: Carbo v.

    White as if dead: Calc.

COLDNESS: Calc., Chel., Con., Sep.

    And deadness; of F. and limbs: Sep.

        Numbness: Con.

    Nails blue from: Nux, Verat.

CONTRACTION: Asa., Graph., *Sec.*

    And numbness: Sec.

    Of F. and toes alt. with spasms of glottis: Asa.

    Spasmodic: Graph.

CRACKING and creaking in joints: Caps.

CRAMPS: Anac., Arn., Ars., Cup., Ferr., Merc., Sec., Stann., Verat.

CRAMPS; In F. of l. hand: Arn.
> Painful: Merc.
> With pains: PLUMB., Verat.

CRAMPLIKE sensation: Mag. c.

CRAWLING: Cham., Rhus, Sec.
> In tips: Rhus, Sec.
> Sensation: Rhus, Sec.
> Tearing: Cham.

CRUMPLES or long furrows in nails: Fluo. ac.

CRUSHED, nails grow in splits if: Ant. c.

DEAD, cold white as if: Calc.

DEADNESS and coldness of F. and limbs: Sep.
> Of one-half, sharply defined: Phos ac.

DISCOLORED, nails become: Graph., Sil., Thuya.

DISPOSITION to felons: DIOS., *Natr. s.*

DRAWING: Acon., *Arn.*, *Bell.*, Canst., Cic., Dig., Hell., Hep., Natr. s., Puls.

DRAWING and tearing in joints: BELL.
> Extending to: Apis.
> In joints of: Bell., Caul., Caust.
>> R. thumb: Arn.
>> Tendons: Caust., Cic.
> Painful, in posterior joint of l. middle: Bell.
> Paralytic: Dig.
> Tearing: Hep., Lyc.. Sulf.
> Up and down: Nux.
> Violent: Hell.
> See also Pain drawing.

ELBOW: See Pain severe.

ENDS, inflammation of: Alum., Amm. c., Fluo. ac., Natr. s.

EXCORIATED, nails: Graph.

EXTENDED, cannot be: Ars., Plumb.

FELON: *Alum.*, Amm. c., Apis, Arn., Bufo, *Dios.*, *Fluo. ac.*, Graph., Hep., NATR. S., Sil., Stram.
> At root of nail, tendency to exuberant granulations: ALUM., Arn., Graph.
> Nail brittle, lancinating pains, tendency to ulceration of F. tips: ALUM.
> See also Pain.

FLEXED, become, and cannot be opened without assistance, even though great exertion be used: MERC.

FLEXORS, great paralysis of: Mez.

FURROWS, long on nails, or crumpled: Fluo. ac.

FUZZY and insensible, F. and toes feel: Sec.

GLOTTIS: See Contractions.

GOUT alt. with gastric troubles: Kali bi.

  Stiff, from: Agar.

GRANULATIONS, tendency to exuberant: *Alum.*, Arn.,
                Graph.

GROWTHS come under nails: Ant. c.

HALF,·deadness sharply defined of one: Phos. ac.

HAND, cramp in F. of l.: Arn.

  Skin peels off between thumb and F. of each: Amm. m.

HEAVINESS and numbness: Phos.

       Of tips: Phos.

HORNY, nails become: Ant. c.

IMPRESSIONS in F., unusually deep, from using scissors
    or other instruments: Bov.

INABILITY to extend or open: PLUMB.

INDEX, paralytic tearing in middle of r. (joint): Bell.·

  See also Pain.

INFLAMMATION at root of nails with tendency to exuberant granulations: ALUM., Arn., Graph.

  Of ends: Alum., Amm. c., Natr. s.

  Redness and swelling of joints: Lyc.

  See also Felons.

INJURED F. looks black, pains streak up arm: Bufo.

INSENSIBLE: Sec., Verat.

INSENSIBILITY of F. and toes with fuzzy feeling: Sec.

JERKING: Ars., China, Fluo. ac., Nitr. s., Phos. ac.

  And burning pains, violent, esp. in index: Fluo. ac.

  Sensation: Natr. c., Phos. ac.

  Tearing: China.

    In metacarpal bones and F.; <touch: China.

  See also Pain jerking.

JOINTS, aching in: Cann. s.

  Burning as from needles in: Berb.

    In first, and phalanges: Zinc.

  Cold, become: Chel.

  Cracking and creaking in: Caps.

  Drawing and tearing in: Bell.

    In: Ars., Bell., Canst., Natr. s.

  Easily put out of: Hep.

  Inflamed red and swollen: Natr. c.

  Jerking sensation in: Natr. c.

  Paralysis of: Calc. p.

JOINTS; Red, hot swelling of: Hep.

 Redness heat and swelling of: Lyc.

 Rheumatic, pressive tearing in first, of r. thumb: Graph.

 Sensation of jerking in: Natr. c.

 Shooting in: Phyt.

 Swelling about, of wrists, knee and index: Lach.

  Redness and inflammation of: Lyc.

  With neuralgia under nails: Berb.

 Swollen and puffy, feel on writing: Bry.

  Become: Calc.

 Tearing in: Bell., Graph., Sil., Zinc., Rhus.

  In first, of phalanges: Zinc.

  Of F. and thumb: Sil.

  Paralytic in r. index, middle of: Bell.

  Rheumatic, pressive, in middle of r. thumb: Graph.

 Yellow and cold, become: Chel.

LIMBS and F. feel cold and dead: Sep.

MOUTH, must roll something between F. or put F. in: Tarent. H.

NAILS; become black: Graph.

  Blue from cold: Nux, *Verat.*

  Brittle, extremely: *Alum.*, Sil., Thuya.

   Rough or yellow: Sil., Thuya.

  Crumpled or long furrows: Fluo. ac.

  Discolored: Graph., Sil., Thuya.

  Horny: Ant. c.

  Rough and yellow: Sil., Thuya.

  Thicker: Graph.

  Yellow: Sil., Thuya.

Bites: Arum. t.

Blue: Acon.

Brittle, lancinating pain, tendency to ulceration of F. tips: ALUM.

 And many white spots: Spig.

Excoriate: Graph.

Furrows, long, or crumpled: Fluo. ac.

Inflammation at root of, with tendency to exuberant granulations: ALUM., Arn., Graph.

Neuralgia under, with swelling of joints: Graph.

Paronychia: Dios.

Splits, grow in as if crushed: Ant. c.

NAILS, Suppuration under: Form.
    See also Pain, Powder.
NEEDLES, burning in joints as from: Berb.
NEURALGIA: See Nails.
NODOSITIES, Arthritic: Clem., Led.
                        Chronic: Amm. p., Ben. ac., Calc.,
                                Guiac., Staph.
NUMBNESS: Abrot., Apis, Caps., Con., Phos., Sec.,
    And coldness: Con. ,
        Contractions: Sec.
        Heaviness of tips: Phos.
        Stiffness: Bufo.
    Esp. of tips: Apis, Phos.
ONYCHIA, simple: Fluo. ac.
OSTEITIS: *Fluo. ac.*, *Hep.*, SIL.
PAIN: Aching: Cann. s., Dios., Thuya.
    Acute, sudden, in ball of r. thumb, extends to
                        shoulder: Cedron.
    Agonizing, in F., toes, wrists and ankles: Act. s.
    Arthritic: ACT. S., Ant. c., Caul., Kali bi.: Led.
    At night: Caul.
    Arms, streak up: Bufo.
    Boring, violent, in first joint of r. with a feeling of
                  stiffness: Led.
    Bruise, as after a; in ball of r. thumb: Cina.
    Bruised, in balls of both thumbs: Arn.
    Burning: Apis, Bufo, Fagop., Fluo. ac.
        And stinging, in felons, with great soreness:
                        Apis.
        Stinging: Apis, Fagop.
        Violent, with jerking, esp. index: Fluo. ac.
    Drawing: Arn., Ars., Bell., Caul., Nitrum, Puls.
        Jerking and tearing, from tips of F. into
                shoulders: Ars.
    Felon, as if a, would form in l. index: Sil.
        >out doors: Natr. s.
        Intolerable, drives one to despair, >suppurat-
                ing: Stram.
        Runs in streaks up arm: Bufo.
        Throbbing, violent or stitches, on pressing nail:
                Fluo. ac.
        Violent, jerking and burning, esp. of index F.:
                Fluo. ac.

PAIN; In balls of both thumbs, as if bruised: Arn.

     After a bruise: Cina.

  F.: Act. s., Agar., Arn., Caul.. Iris. Led.

  Single F.: Calc. p.

  Jerking: Ars., Fluo.ac., Phos. ac.

    See burning, drawing.

  JOINTS: ACT. S., Arn., Bell., Caul., Cim.. Kali
    bi.. Led.. Phyt., Pip. m., Sep.. Sticta.

    Arthritic: Act. s., Ant. c.

    In l. thumb,<pressure: Pip. m.

  Nail, at root: Alum., Arn.. Graph.

    See throbbing.

  Paralytic, in thumb: Acon.

  Pressing, in r. joints of ring and middle: Arn.

  Pressive. in joints: Arn.

  Severe, from little. along ulna. to elbow: Kalm.

  Sharp, shooting in thumb: Dulc.

  Sprain. as from a. in: Natr. m.

  Sprained, as if. in l. thumb: *Kreos.*. Sec.

  Sticking: Bry., Natr. m.. Sil.

    In. when writing: Bry.

    Jerks, outward. ending in itching. burning:
        Lith. c.

  Stinging. burning: Apis. Fagop.

  Streaking up arm: Bufo.

  Tearing, drawing: Acon., Arn.. *Bell.*

    Extending to F. on motion: Acon.

  Tensive: Iod., Sep.

    Of metacarpal joints: Sep.

  With cramp: PLUMB.. Verat.

  Throbbing. on pressing nail. violent. or sharp
      stitches: Fluo. ac.

PAINFUL cramp: Merc.

  Joints: Ars.

  Soreness: *Eup.*, *perf.*

  See Drawing.

PANARITIUM: See Felon and Pain.

PARALYTIC: See Drawing. Tearing. and Pain.

PARALYSIS, great of flexors: Mez.

  Of joints: Calc. p.

PERIOSTEUM of phalanges. painful on pressure: Led.

PINCHING: See Pricking.

PINS, feel as if, sticking in tips and palmer surface of
　　　first phalanges when grasping anything: Rhus.
PRESSING and Tearing in: Arn., Indigo.
PRICKING in: RHUS.
　　　Or pinching, insensible to, ends horny and thickened:
　　　　　　　　　　　　　　　　　Populus c.
POWDER, nails gray, dirty as if decayed, when cut
　　　scattering like, and splitting into layers: Sil.
REDNESS, inflammation and swelling of joints: Lyc.
RED, hot swelling of joints: *Hep.*
RHAGADES: Bals. p.
RHEUMATIC, pressive tearing in first joint of r. thumb:
　　　　　　　　　　　　　　　　　Graph.
RHEUMATISM: ACT. S., Agar., Ant. c., Bell., Berb,.
　　　Bry., Calc., *Caul.*, China, Ferr., Graph., KALI
　　　BI., Kalm., Kreos., LED., Lyc., Merc., Mez.,
　　　Natr.c., Pip. m., *Rhus*, Sep., Sil., Staph.,*Sulf.*,
　　　Zinc.

　　Of F. and wrist joints: Caul.
　　　Index, and wrists: Lach.
　　　L.: Bell., Kalm., Kreos., Led., Pip. m., Rhus,
　　　　　　　　　　　　　　　　　Sec.

　　　R.: Arn., Bell., Bry., Led., Lyc.
RHEUMATOID arthritis: Calc.
RIGID, easily become: Merc.
ROLL: See Must.
ROUGH, nails become brittle and: Sil., Thuya.
SCISSORS: See Impressions.
SENSATION in tips as if suppurating: Sil.
　　　　　Of jerking in joints: Natr. c.
　　　　　　Numbness: Abrot., Con., Phos., Sec.
SHOOTING in joints: Phyt.
SIMPLE onychia: Fluo. ac.
SKIN peels off between thumb and forefinger of each hand:
　　　　　　　　　　　　　　　　　Amm. m.
SPASMODIC contractions: Graph.
SPLITS, nails grow in, if crushed: Ant. c.
SPRAINED, stiff pain in l. thumb: Kreos.
SPREAD apart or bent backward, are fingers and toes:
　　　　　　　　　　　　　　　　　Sec.
STICKING: Bry., Cann. s., Natr. s., Sulf.
　　　　In bones of little: Cann. s.
　　　　　Tips: Pet., Sulf.

STIFF from gout: Agar.

STIFFNESS: Caul., Ferr., Hep.

> Feeling of, with boring in first joint of r. thumb: Led.

> Sudden: Dig.

STITCHES: Bry., Kali c., Phos. ac., Val.

SWELLING: Berb., *Bry.*, Bufo, Calc., Hep., Lyc., *Rhus*.

> Of joints with neuralgia under nails: Berb.

> Red, hot: Hep.

> Redness and inflammation: Hep.

SWOLLEN and puffed, joints feel, on writing or taking hold of anything, painful on touch, or exertion: Bry.

> Feel as if, but no visible swelling: Calc.

> Joints become: Calc.

TEARING and pressing: Arn., Indigo.

> In back of: Natr. c.

> First joints of phalanges: Zinc.

> Index: Zinc.

> Joints: Calc., Rhus.

> > Of F. and thumb: Sil.

> Thumb: Agar., Graph.

> Jerking, in metacarpal bones and F, <touch: China.

> Paralytic, in middle joint of r. index: Bell.

> Rheumatic pressive, in first joint of r. thumb: Graph.

THICKER, nails become: Graph.

THUMB, boring in first joint of r. with a feeling of stiffness: Led.

> Drawing in: Arn.

> Tearing in: Agar., Graph., Sil.

> > Joints of F. and: Sil.

> > Rheumatic, pressive, in first joint of r.: Graph.

> See also Pain and Skin.

TINGLING in skin: Acon.

TIPS, crawling in: Rhus, Sec.

> Heaviness and numbness of: Phos.

> Sticking in: Pet., Sulf.

> Suppurating sensation in: Sil.

> Sweat covered with cold: Carbo v.

TIRED and ache when writing: Fagop.

TOES: See Spread.

TREMBLE when writing: *Cim.*

ULNA: See Pain severe.

VIOLENT drawing in: Hell.

          Twitching extending to: Arn.

WHITE, cold as if dead: Calc.

WHITLOW: See Felon.

WRITING, joints feel swollen and puffed while: Bry.

          Tremble while: *Cim.*

          See Pain Sticking.

YELLOW, become cold and: Chel.

# SPINE, CORD AND VERTEBRAE.

ABDOMEN: See Pain cutting.

ANAEMIA, spinal: China, Dig., Phos.

    From seminal emissions: Calc., China, Dig., Phos ac.

    Palpitation, impotency and pain in vertex, from sexual excesses: Phos. ac.

ANTS, sensation of, creeping along S.: Agar.

ARMS, cries from slightest motion of, or neck after a fall: Hyperic.

ATAXIA, locomotor: Phos., Plumb., Stram., Thall., Zinc.

    And progressive S. paralysis: Phos.

    Early stages of: Gels., Stram.

    First stage of: Gels.

    Limbs unsteady, lightning like pains: Plumb.

    See Neuralgia and Pain.

ATROPHY, S., progressive muscular: Ars., Plumb.

    With sciatic pains: Plumb.

BACKWARD, S. bent and stiff: Petr.

BAND, feeling of a tight, around body (Cact., Lyc.), in caries of V.: Phos.

BODY, S. feels too weak to support: Arn.

    Twitching of, uncommon, in S. irritation: Ambra.

  See Band.

BROKEN, S. seems as if: Cina.

BRUISED, muscles feel as if during S. congestion: Gels.

  See Pain bruised.

BRUISES, ill effects of, to S.: Con.

BURNING: Agar., Bell., Hell., Phos.. Pic. ac.

    And stinging of C.: Agar., (Apis).

    In S. marrow: Bell.

        With headache and diarrhœa: Pic. ac.

    Of S. processes: Phos.

    Sensation as if S. marrow was on fire: Bell.

    Spots in S.: Agar.

BURNING; Stitches in region of S.: Hell.
See also Pain burning.
CARIES of lumbar V.: Phos. ac.
V. cannot bear heat to back (Agar.), feeling of a tight band around body (Cact., Lyc.):
Phos.
CHEST, oppression of, with sensitiveness of last cervical and upper dorsal V.: China, Hyperic.
CHOREA; Attacks crosswise: Agar., Stram., Tarent. H. Upper r. and lower l. or vice versa: Agar.
During sleep: Zinc,, Zizia.
With fidgety feet: Zinc.
Legs: Zizia
From a cold bath: Rhus.
Of r. arm and l. leg, which are constantly in motion.
Cannot do anything; attacks preceded by malaise: Tarent. H.
Nocturnal, of children: Tarent. H.
S.: Nux.
Unaffected by sleep: Verat.
With constant movements of limbs, esp. hands: Tarent.
Twitchings, which continue during sleep: Opi.
COCCYX. stiffness of V. beginning in, and going up to nape of neck: Ars.
COLDNESS along V. column: Acon.
And uncommon twitching, with irritation of S.: Ambra.
CONCUSSION of S. after a fall, cries from slighest touch or motion of arms or neck: Hyperic.
CONVULSIONS, tendency to, from injuries to S.: Zinc.
COÖRDINATION, hyperæmia with loss of, when walking: *Bell.*, Gels.
CORD, burning, stinging in: *Agar.*, (Apis).
Painfulness of, when stooping: Agar.
Softening of: Crotal. h., Phos.
COUGH from pressure on dorsal V.: Bell.
With gnawing in S.: Bell.
CRACKING of V.: Aloe, Chel., Natr. c., Niccol., Sulf.
Cervical V. on turning head: Natr. c., Niccol., Sulf.

CREEPING along S, as from ants: Agar.

CURVATURE of S.: Calc. c. and p., Lyc., Phos., Sulf., Thuya.

    Abscess and emaciation: Sil.

    Stands bent forward: Thuya.

    V. soften: Phos., Sulf.

CUTTING from S. to abdomen in a circle: Acon.

    In umbilicus and lumbar V.: Rheum.

    Stitching, pulsating, as if a' portion of S. had been taken out: Natr. m.

DIARRHŒA and headache with burning in S.: Pic. ac.

DISTORTION of V. column, with commencing paraplegia: Tarent.

DORSAL region sensitive to pressure: China, Cim.

    Tenderness of on pressure: Plumb.

    V., esp. last, sensitive to touch: Zinc.

    First, and last cervical, sensitive to pressure: Chin. s.

DRAWING, tearing, in and S.: Caps.

    Through lumbar V.: Con.

    See also Pain drawing.

DULL pressure in both sides of V.: Colch.

    Stitches in and near S.: Hell.

GNAWING in S., with cough: Bell.

HEAD, last cervical and first dorsal V. sensitive to pressure, pain extends to: Chin. s.

HEART: See Pressure in.

HEAT, dry, with S. irritation: Sulf.

HEMIPLEGIA following vertigo: Oleand.

INJURIES, tendency to convulsions from, to S.: Zinc.

IRRITABLE S.: Agar., Bell.

    Pressure on dorsal V. causes either screams and distress in stomach or violent cough and flushed face: Bell.

IRRITABLE, weak S.: Agar.

IRRITATION of S.: Ambra, Calc., Cup., Nux, Petr., Sulf.

    From sexual excesses: Calc., Nux.

    Limbs go to sleep easily: Nux, Petr.

    Violent paroxysms of pain, S. extremely sensitive: Cup.

    With suppressed menses or hæmorrhoids, with dry heat: Sulf.

IRRITATION of S. with uncommon twitching and coldness of body: Ambra.

Weakness of chest and stomach and sleeplessness: Sulf.

LIMBS: See Ataxia and S. irritation.

LOCOMOTOR ataxia: See Ataxia.

LUMBAR V., caries of: Phos. ac.

MENINGITIS: Arn., Dulc., Hyperic.

S. during scarlet fever and measles, when rash does not appear: Dulc.

Traumatic, cerebro-S.: Arn., Hyperic.

MYELITIS after taking cold: Dulc.

NECK: See Concussion and Coccyx.

NEURALGIA of S. (6th. cervical V.), extends up and down to shoulders, with weight, numbness and heat; soreness on top of head so that he could not brush his hair, eyelids heavy: Paris.

In locomotor ataxia: Agar.

Starts between shoulders, with tenderness over S., and pain in occiput: Ox. ac.

PAIN: Across shoulders and S.: Cann. i.

Acute, in region of lumbar V.: Glon.

Beaten, as if, in S.: Ruta.

Bruised, in lumbar V.: Hep.

Burning, shooting, deep in S.: Agar.

Cardialgic with tired feeling in S. and shoulders: *Arg. n.*, Verat.

Constant, in S.: Kalm.

Cutting, in a circle, from S. to abdomen: Acon.

Drawing, from pubic region to middle of S.: Plumb.

In middle of S.: Stram.

Tearing, down whole S.: Cina.

Near S.: Caps.

Tensive, at points of cervical and upper dorsal V.: China, *Cim.*, Sulf.

Extends from S. to head.: China, Chin. s., Hyperic.

Periodically: Chin. s.

In all V. as if sore: Chel.

Chest, caused by slightest touch of S: Tarent. H.

Curved S.: Sil.

Lower half of S. column and sacrum: Thuya.

Neck, as if in cervical V.: Carbo v.

Occiput, with neuralgia of S.: Ox. ac.

PAIN; in remote parts from pressure on S.: Sil.

    S., as if it would break: Coccul.

    S. Caused every motion or turn of body: Agar.

    Stomach, with tired feeling in S.: *Arg. n.*, Bell.

Intense at night, in S., with trembling: Tarent. H.

In upper cervical V.: Chel.

    Dorsal V. at points of S. processes: *Cim.*

Jerking, tearing, in middle of S.: Cina.

Lancinating: Ginseng.

Lightninglike: Cim., Mag., Plumb., Zinc.

    Violent in posterior sclerosis: *Cim.*

Neuralgic, violent, in paralysis: Plumb.

On both sides of S.: Ox. ac.

Paroxysms of terrible, screams if S. is touched: Hyperi.

Piercing, in articulations of V.: Coccul.

Pinching, in middle of S.: Phos. ac.

    Pressive, near lowest portion of S.: Carbo v.

Radiate from dorsal S. and meet over stomach and abdomen (Acon.): Mag. p.

Running down S.: Phyt.

Sciatic, violent, in paralysis: Plumb.

    In progressive muscular atrophy: Plumb.

Severe, bruised, in S.: Mag. m.

Shooting, burning, deep in S.: Agar.

    In V.: Agar.

Sore, in all V., as if: Chel.

Sticking in S.: Euphr., Ign.

    Violent: Euphra.

Stinging and burning in C.: Agar., (Apis.)

    With soreness of S., could not tell when foot touched ground: Apis.

Tearing, in S.: Cina, Lyc., Natr. m.

    Jerking, in middle of S.: *Cina.*

Terrible: See paroxysms.

Violent, in S.: Arn., Chel., Cup., Lalm., Phos., Plumb., Thall.

    After writing: Arn.

    Long stooping, as: Arn.

In locomotor ataxia: Plumb., Thall.

    Lumbar V.: Chel.

    Upper third of dorsal V.: Kalm.

PAIN; Violent in V. column: Phos.

               Sticking, along whole S.: Euphra.

PAINFUL pressure in middle of S.: Arn.

             Stitches in middle of S.: Dulc.

PAINFULNESS along C.: *Agar.*

          Of C. when stooping: Agar.

           S. at every turning motion: Agar.

          On lying down: Natr. m.

PARALYSIS: *Acon.*, Agar., Apis, Bar. c., Cann. i., *Caust.*,
        Cup., Curare, Hyos., Mag., LED., *Merc.*,
            Phos., PLUMB., RHUS, Zinc.

Acute ascending from periphery to cord: Con.

Agitans: Hyos., Mag. p.

      After spasms: Hyos.

PARALYSIS; Ascending: Con., Led., Sulf.

Commencing in lower limbs and traveling upward:
              Con., Led., Sulf.

         Upper limbs and traveling downward:
                  Merc.

Complete: PLUMB., ACET.

     Of upper and lower, or vice versa: Con.

     Or partial, with drawing pains: PLUMB.
                      ACET.

Convulsive movements of groups of muscles, preceed:
    Coccul.

Following apoplexia: Bar. c., Guaco.

           In old age: Bar. c.

      Epileptic attacks: Curare.

      Rachitic curvature of S.: Phos.

From cerebro-S. softening: Pic. ac.

    Cold, dry winds: Acon., Canst.

      Drenching rain: Phos., Rhus.

           Feels as if quicksilver moved up
              and down S.: Phos.

      Fright, internal, externally cold: Cup.

      Getting wet: Dulc., Phos., RHUS.

           Or lying on damp ground: Dulc.,
                  RHUS.

               Parts stiff and
               numb: RHUS.

Hemiplegia: Oleand.

Of flexors: Cup, Plumb., Sec.

    Limbs, cramps, numbness and formication: (Acon.)
                      Sec.

PARALYSIS of lower extremities: Agar., Cann. i., Con., Led., Merc., Phos., Plumb., Sulf.

And upper: Agar., Phos., Plumb.

R. arm: Cann. i.

One side, convulsions of the other: Apis, Bell.

Upper: See lower.

Painful, after apoplexia: Guaco.

Partial, legs cold and bluish: Nux.

Progressive S., and locomotor ataxia: Phos.

Rheumatic: Nitrum, Plumb., *Rhus*.

S.: Plumb.

With numbness and tingling alt. with articular pains: Nitrum.

Symptoms of, esp. with anaemia, hands seem cold and numb: Graph.

Menses disordered, limbs numb: Puls.

Ol l. hand and l. leg, hand feels dead when sewing: Crot. h.

Violent neuralgic and sciatic pains with: PLUMB.

With coldness, numbness (Sec.) and tingling: Acon.

Drawing pains: Plumb. acet.

Lightninglike pains: Plumb., Zinc.

Rickets: Phos., Sil.

PLUG, feeling of a, in S.: Anac.

POTTS' disease: Calc. p., Merc. corr., Sil.

Abscess, curvature and emaciation: Sil.

<nights, no >from sweats: Merc. corr.

PRESSURE and stitches in region of S.: Nitrum.

In S. and stomach alt. with violent beating of heart: Bism.

On S. caused pain in remote parts: Sil.

Spinous processes sensitive to: Agar., Phos.

PULSATING, cutting stitching, as if a portion of S. had been taken out: Natr. m.

RHEUMATIC drawing from upper dorsal V.: Euphra.

RICKETS with paralysis: Phos., Sil.

SENSATION as if ice touched S. marrow: Agar.

Of ants crawling along S.: Agar.

SENSITIVE, last cervical and first dorsal V., to pressure, oppression of chest, pain extends to head and is periodical: Chin. s.

Remarkably, along S., in cervical region: Stram.

SENSITIVE, S., esp. cervical and dorsal (upper) region, to pressure: China, Chin. s., Cim.

Extremely so, to touch, pains extend to head: China, Chin. s., *Hyperic.*

Its whole length, with violent paroxysms of pain: Cup.

To touch, esp. last dorsal V ,, <sitting still and stimulants: Zinc.

SENSITIVENESS along s.: Stram.

Great between V.: Therid.

SHOCKS, ill effect of to S.: Con.

SHOOTING and gnawing in S. column: Bell.

SORE, See Pain sore.

SORENESS of S.: See Pain stinging.

Processes: Phos.

SPINAL anaemia from sexual excesses: Phos. ac:

Seminal emissions: Dig., China,

Chorea: Nux.                                    Phos. ac.

See Meningitis.

SPINE bent backward and stiff: Petr.

Painful when walking: Verat.

SPINUS processes sensitive to pressure: Agar., Phos.

Sore: Phos.

STIFFNESS in S.: Ars., Nitr. c.

See Coccyx.

STITCHES and pressure in region of S.: Nitrum.

Burning, in region of S.: Hell.

Painful in middle of S.: Dulc.

STITCHING: See pulsating.

STOMACH: See Irritation and Pain in.

TEARING in cervical V.: Lach.

Fear S.: Lyc.

TENDERNESS of S., paroxysms of terrible pain, screaming if approached: Hyperic.

TENSION in dorsal V.: Canst.

TIRED: See Pain in.

TOUCH, S. sensitive to: *Agar.*, Arn.. China, Cim., *Phos.*

TRAUMATIC cerebro-S., meningitis: Arn., Hyperic.

VERTEBRAE, softening in S., curvature of: Phos., Suls.

VERTIGO followed by hemiplegia: Oleand.

WALKING, hyperameia of S., with loss of coordination when: Bell., (Gels.).

WEAK, irritable S.: Agar.

# BACK.

ABDOMEN, burning in, with cold sweat on B. and breast:
Cub.

Cold with B. ache: Sarsap.

Plethoric with B. ache: Nux.

ACHING: AESC., Apis, Calc., Cann. i., CIM., Helon.,
Nux, Puls.

And colic at same time: Sarsap.

Constant: Aesc., *Cann. i.*

No$>$nor$<$: Cann. i.

Dull: Caul.

In liver extending through whole dorsal region: Polyp.

Mostly between shoulder blades: Calc. p.

Of,$>$pressure: Natr. m.

Or pain in posterior aspect of spleen: Lob. c.

Tensive: Hep.

Tired, in B. and legs, excessive fatigue and burning
in dorsal region: Helon.

Very severe when moving: Aesc., Bry.

With abdominal plethora: Nux.

Coldness of abdomen: Sarsap.

Constipation and piles: Euonym.

Uterine pains: Calc. p., *Cim.*, Puls.

ARCH, B. bent backward like an: Absinth., *Cic.*, Cup.,
Nux, Oenanth., OPI., *Cim.*

Curved like an, from violent trembling motion of
limbs: Opi.

APART, B. and limbs feel as if falling,$>$tight bandaging: Trill.

BENT: See Arch.

BOARD, B. feels like a, and painfully stiff: Puls.

As if lying on a: ARV., Bapt.

BODY, B. feels to weak to support,$>$change of position,
$<$thinking of it, pain extends down thighs
(Cim., Nit. ac.): Ox. ac.

BROKEN, B. feels as if: Carbo an., *Kali c.*, *Gossyp.*,
Natr. m., OVA T.

BROKEN, B. feels as if and tied with a string: OVA T.

Cannot lie on it, must lie on stomach: Gossyp.

On walking, standing or lying: Carbo an.

BRUISED, muscles of B. feel: Agar., ARN., Eup. perf.

Sensation in muscles of B. and loins: Cham., Eup. perf.

Pressive, in B. and loins, early on rising, $<$ turning trunk or standing, $>$ walking: Thuya.

BURNING: Cub., Helon., *Lyc.*, Merc., *Nux*, Pic. ac., *Sil.*, Tereb.

Heat in dorsal region: Helon.

While walking in open air and becoming warm: Sil.

See also Abdomen and Pain burning.

CHEST, stitches shooting to, from B.: Bry.

CHILLS begin in B., with severe pains: Caps.

In B.: Gels.

Running over B.: Apis.

COLD water, shivering over B. as if, were being poured over it, with heat of face: Anac.

Sensation of, dropping down B.: Caps.

On or from B.: Cann. s.

COLDNESS in B.: Sec.

Of glutii: Calc., Agar.

Sudden feeling of: Croc. s.

CONSTANT throbbing: Lyr.

See Pain constant.

CONTRACTIONS and stiff neck, with rheumatic pains in muscles of B.: China, *Cim.*, Clem., Dulc.

CRAMP and pain in loins and B.: Bell.

In B.: Bell., Dros.. Petr.

CRICK in: *Acon.*, Agar.

Extends to nape of neck: *Agar.*

CURVED: See Arch.

DORSAL region, burning heat in: Helon.

DRAWING in: Ars., Cham., Natr. m., Thuya.

Middle of: Stram.

Tearing, pressing, sticking in: Cham.

See Pain drawing.

DROPPING; See Cold water.

DULL B. ache: Caul.

See also Pain dull.

FORMICATION in: Sec.

GLUTII, coldness of: *Agar.*, Calc.

HEAD, heat in, extends down b.: Cim.

HEAT: See Aching tired and Head.

HEAVINESS, Carbo. v., Petr.

    See Pain dull.

HIPS: See Apart and Pain.

HYPERÆSTHESIA, excessive: Tarent. H.

INTERMITTING violent stitches: Euphorb.

KINK in B. hindering deep inspiration: Acon.

KNEES drawn up, lies on B.: Merc. corr.

    See Weakness of.

LAME, B. and limbs sore and, <A. M.: Agar., Rhus.

    In region of liver: Dios.

LAMENESS (Calc., Natr. m., Rhus.), stiffness (Rhus) and weight, with pain in B.: Helon.

LASSITUDE: Ginseng.

LEGS: See Aching tired.

LIE, must on stomach, cannot on B.: Gossyp.

        B.: Anac.

LIES on B.: Ambra, Anac., Merc. corr.

    With knees drawn up: Merc. corr.

LIMBS: See Arch and Lame.

LIVER: See Aching and pain.

LOAD, sensation as if a, would drop from pit of stomach to B.: Lauro.

LYING on B.. <uterine pains: Ambra.

    See Board, Broken.

MUSCLES painful: Tarent. H.

   Rigid: Stram.

       Of B. and neck: Caul.

NECK: See Crick and Stiffness.

NETTLES, stitches or stinging in B. as from: Caust.

NIPPLE: See Pain from.

OUT, B. gives, when walking: AESC., Kali c.

PAIN; Aching: *Aesc., Calc., Cim.*, Nux, Puls., *Rhus.*

    Acute: Glon.

    Agonizing in B. and hips: Arn.

    Beaten, as if: Stann., Stram., Sulf., Zinc.

    Broken, as if: Natr. m., OVA T., Phos., *Plat.*

    Bruise and sprain, as from a: Agar., Arn., China, Eup. Perf., Merc.

PAIN; Bruised: Apis, Berb., Eup. perf., *Kali c.*, Merc.,
　　　　　Nux, Psor., *Zinc.*

　　　As if: Arn., Merc.
　　　　　From stooping: Cham.
　　　During rest: Kali c.
　　　From stooping: Cham.
　　　While walking in open air: Zinc.
　　　With stiffness in B., rises from a seat with
　　　　　　difficulty: Berb.
　Burning, sticking: Calc., Verat.
　　　Tearing: Nux.
　Colicky, extends to B.: Bism., Dios., Nux, Plat.
　Constant, and bruised sensation: Nux.
　　　Pressive: Euphra.
　Cramp and, in loins and B.: Bell.
　Drawing in B.: *Cham.*, Thuya.
　　　While sitting: Thuya.
　Dull: Caul.
　　Heavy: Bolet.
　Excoriating, extorting cries and causing him to
　　　　double up, during chill: Caps.
　Extends to B.: *Berb.*, Bism., Carbo v., Caust., Chel.,
　　　　*Dios.*, Crot. t., Nux, Plat.
　From nipple to B. as from a string: Crot. t.
　　　Stomach to B., and vice versa: Berb.
　Hard: Dios.
　Heavy, dull: Bolet.
　In B. and r. side, from congestion of liver: Lyc.
　　　With stiffness, lameness and weight: Helon.
　　Dorsal and lumbar regions, constant sexual excite-
　　　　ment, severe erections, (Pic. ac.), numbness
　　　　and tingling (Acon.) in feet and legs: Onos.
　　Liver, extending to B. and shoulders: Chel.
　　Middle of B.: Cann. s.
　　Muscles of B.: GUIAC., Plumb.
　Jerking, Sticking: Euphorb.
　Lying on something hard, >from: Natr. m.
　Making walking difficult: Bry.
　Muscular, with stiffness: Guiac.
　On riding in a carriage: Nux m.
　　Stooping: Sulf.
　Or aching in posterior aspect of spleen: Lob. c.
　Over shoulder blades: Apis.

PAIN; Rheumatic: Bell., Cim., Dulc., Kali.c.

    In muscles of B.: Acon., China, *Cim.,* Cham., Dulc.

    And neck, with stiffness contraction: China, *Cim.,* Dulc.

Severe in B., through hips and down thighs: *Cim.,* Nitr. ac., Ox. ac.

Severe, with chill: Caps.

Sharp, cutting, drawing: Cup.

Shooting: Sil.

Soreness and: Sep.

Spasmodic, in liver, extends to B. and shoulders: Chel., Ferr.

Sticking: Stann., Zinc.

Stitching, extending into gluteal muscles: Kali c.

Stomach, from B. to, before menses: Borax.

Stooping, as after: Agar., *Dulc.,* Graph.

    In B. on: Sulf.

Tearing: Canth., Sil.

    Arthritic: Sil.

Uterine, with B. ache: Calc. p., Cim., Puls.

Violent, as if sprained: Caust.

    Bruised on sitting, goes off on motion:
    Down B.: Kalm.         [Rhus.

    In B.: Digitalin, Rhus, Tongo.

    Very: Digitalin.

Walking, after: Phos.

Wandering: Chel., Puls.

Wearied by too great effort, as if: Zinc.

Wrenched, as if: Calc.

Urinating, > after: Lyc.

With stiffness, lameness and weight: Helon.

PAINFUL stiffness in when stooping: Cic.

PARALYZED feeling in extremities and weakness in B.: Sil.

PINCHING and drawing in B.: Lyc.

PRESSIVE bruised sensation in B. and loins, early on rising, < on turning trunk, standing or walking:

PRESSURE: Lyc., PETR.

RHEUMATIC drawing in B.: Carbo v.

RHEUMATISM: Acon., Calc., Cim., Dulc., Nux, RHUS.
Of B. and Hips: Phyt.

SENSATION as if bruised in muscles of B. and loins: Cham., Eup. perf.

See also Cold and Load.

SHIVERING: See Cold.

SHOULDERS: See Pain spasmodic.

SITTING, sticking in B. and small of B., while, and walking: Zinc.

See also Pain drawing and violent.

SORE, bruised sensation: Thuya.

SORENESS: Rhus, Sep., Thuya.

And lameness of B. and limbs, <A. M.: Agar., Rhus.

Pain: Sep.

Weakness: Pic. ac.

SPLEEN: See Pain or.

STANDING, weight in B. when: Arg. n.

See Broken.

STICKING in B.: Lach., Lyc., Nitr. ac., Zinc.

And small of B. while sitting and walking: Zinc.

STIFFNESS: *Acon.*, Berb., *Calc.*, Carbo an., China, Cic., Cim., Clem., Dulc., Guiac., Led., Puls., RHUS.

And lameness: Helon., *Kali c.*

And weight: Helon.

Excessive, of one side, from neck to small of B.: Guiac.

Extending down B.: Lyc.

Up B.: Ars.

Great, every morning: Phyt.

In B. between shoulders: Cic., *Chel.*

Painful, like a board: Puls.

With muscular pains: Guiac.

See also Pain bruised and rheumatic.

STITCHES or stinging as from nettles: Caust.

Shooting from B. to chest: Bry.

STOMACH: See Lie, Load, Pain from.

STOOPING: See Pain stooping.

STRING: See Broken and Pain from.

SWEAT: See Abdomen.

TEARING: Nux, Petr., Phos. ac., Sil.

THIGHS: See Body and Pain severe.

THROBBING: Sil.

TIGHTENED feeling: Mag. c.

TIRED: See Aching.

TREMBLING: Coccul.

    And weakness: Cim.

URINATING>B.: Lyc.

UTERINE pains with B. ache: Calc. p., *Cim.*, Puls.

    Symptoms<lying on B.: Gossyp.

WALKING, B. gives out when: AESC., *Kali c.*

    See also Broken, Pain bruised and Sticking.

WATER: See cold.

WEAK: See Body.

WEAKNESS: Dig., Dios., Nux, Sil.

    And soreness: Pic. ac.

    Of B. and knees after seminal emissions:
Dig., Dios.

    Paralyzed feeling in lower extremities: Sil.

WEARINESS: Clem., Sil.

WEIGHT, lameness, stiffness and pain: Helon.

    When standing: Arg. n.

# SCAPULAR REGION.

ACHING: *Aesc.*, Ail., Cina, Merc., Natr. m., *Sep.*
        Beneath: Merc., Natr. m., Sep.
        Between: *Aesc.*, Ail., *Sep.*
            Dull: Aesc.
            Great, and under l. (Ail.; Chel., Chen.;
                r.) extending into l. lung: Sep.
      In, on motion: Cina.
BACK: See Pain.
BORING and bruised feeling: Mag. m.
BRUISED: See Pain bruised.
BURNING as from glowing coals: Lyc.
        Between: *Lyc.*, Phos.. Zinc.
        Spot between, >rubbing: Phos.
        Violent: Mag. m.
        See also Pain burning.
CHEST: See Pain in and severe.
COALS: See burning.
COLD water, feeling of: Abies c.
      Wind blowing on, sensation of: Caust.
COLDNESS as from a piece of ice on: Led.
        Icy: Amm. m., Natr. m.
CRAMP in: Phos.
DRAWING in: Berb.
            And below: Natr. s.
        Pressure: Kali c.
        Tearing: Acon.
        See also Pain drawing.
DULL aching: Aesc.
      Stitches in l., return slowly and radiate in all direc-
                tions: Anac.
      See also Pain dull.
HEART: See Pain Lancinating.
ICE, feels as if a piece lay between: Lachn.
        See also Coldness.

ICY coldness in: Amm. m., Natr. m.

LAMENESS and stiffness of: Dulc.

LUNG: See Aching between.

NECK: See Pain rheumatic.

PAIN: Aching: *Aesc.*, Ail., Cina, Merc., Nat. m., Sep.

  Across: Ars., Cann. i.

  　Preventing walking erect *Cann. i.*

  And stitches beneath r.: Chel.

  　Tearing: Berb., Caust.

  Bruised: Acon., Dig., Graph.

  　In and on: Aloe.

  　Sprained: Amm. m.

  Burning, sticking: Calc.

  Constant, also stitches, beneath lower angle of r.
  　(Ab. c., Chel., Chen.; l. Ail.): Pod.

  　In, and down back: Sep.

  Contractive: Graph.

  Drawing: Calc., Col., Lyc., *Sulf.*

  　Internally in r.: Col.

  　Tearing: Acon.

  Dull: Hell.

  In: Amm. c., Bell., Caps., Cim., Hep., Naja,
  　Nitr. ac., *Nux.*, Puls., *Rhus. Verat.*

  　As from a strain: Bell.

  　If hurt or sprained: Carbo an.

  　And most below: *Calc. p.*

  　R. and chest: Aesc.

  　With colic: Amm. c., Nitr. ac.

  Lancinating: Ginseng., Glon.

  　From heart to: Glon.

  　Severe, and stitches below r., >throw-
  　　ing shoulders back or chest
  　　forward: Bad.

  Muscular, at lower margin of S., in sedentary
  　women, from long continued sewing or writ-
  　　　ing *Ran. bulb.*, Zinc.

  Over: Apis.

  Piercing, as of knives: Natr. s.

  Rheumatic: Bell., Bry., *Dios.*, Mez., Nux, RHUS,
  　　Staph., *Verat.*

  　In, extends from nape of neck to small
  　　L.: Lyc.　　　　　　　　　　[of back:

PAIN; Rheumatic in Muscules, like a tension and as if
                swollen, making motion difficult:
                                              Mez.
                Very severe: Colch.
                Violent, neither>nor<by rest, but>
                        warmth<cold: Rhus.
        Severe, behind: Phyt.
                In inner angle of r. lower, runs to chest
                (Chel., runs from chest.): Aphis chen.
        Sprained, bruised: Amm. m.
                Or hurt, as if: Carbo an.
        Sticking, and stitches: Chel.
                Under: Aloe.
        Strain, as from a: Bell.
        Stunning: Cann. i.
        Tearing: Petr., Sil.
                In l.: Oleand.
                Violent in and beneath: Sil.
        Tensive, while lying or moving: Sulf.
        Throbbing, in a small spot: Phos.
        Under l.: Ail., Cim.
                R.: Ab. c., CHEL., Chenop., Pod.
                Violent: Digitalin.
PAINFUL sensation on inner surface: Cic.
        Stiffness: *Led.*
        Tension: Carbo an., Cic.
                Of inner surface: Cic.
PRESSURE and drawing in: Bry.
                Oppression in r. extends through to
                        sternum: Chel.
                Tension beneath: Con.
        In: Calc.
        On motion, impeding respiration: Calc.
        Violent, as if bruised; Verat. a.
RHEUMATISM: *Acon.*, *Bry.*, Merc., Mez., *Nux.*, RHUS,
                                              Verat.
SENSATION of cold wind blowing on: Caust.
                Stiffness and weakness of, extending to
                        neck: Agar.
SEWING: See Pain muscular.
SPINOUS processes, as if sore: Phos.
SPOT, burning in a.>rubbing: Phos.
        See Pain throbbing.
STERNUM, pressure and oppression in r., extends to: Chel.

STIFFNESS: Agar., Chel., Dulc., Led., Lyc.

    And Lameness across: Dulc.

      Weakness, sensation of, extending to
              neck: Agar.

    'Extending down back: Lyc.

    Painful: Led.

STITCHES: See Dull, Pain constant and sticking.

TEARING in: Agar., Mag. m., Psor.

    See Pain tearing.

TENSION, painful: Carbo an.

        Of inner surface: Cic.

VIOLENT stitch beneath: Colch.

WATER, feeling of cold, on: Ab. c.

WIND, sensation of cold, blowing: Caust.

---

# RENAL REGION.

ACHING: *Eup. purp.*, Hydrast. Zingib.

    And hot sensation in l.: Zingib.

    Dull: Hydrast.

    In, and bladder, with dysurea: Eup. purp.

      Both, with frequent desire to urinate: Zingib.

BACK: See Pain cramplike and pressive, Soreness.

BAND of clothes causes pain in: Chel.

BLADDER: See Aching, Burning in, Stitches.

BODY: See Tired feeling.

BRUISED sore sensation: Thuya.

BURNING: Berb., Tereb.

    And soreness: Berb.

     Dull pain: Tereb.

    In, and bladder before and during urination:
                Rheum.

    See also Pain burning.

CHEST: See Pain in.

CHILLINESS: See Pain darting.

CLOUDINESS: See Pain in.

COLD: See Pain in.

DULL: See Aching and Pain dull.

DRISTESS in, great: Lact. ac.

HEAT and tension: Natr. m.

HICCOUGH: See Pain burning.

HOT sensation in l. and dull aching: Zingib.

ILLIUM: See Pain agonizing.

KNIVES: See Pain in.

LAMENESS: See Pain in.

LIFTING: See Pain in.

LOINS: See Pain in.

NOSE: See Pain in.

PAIN; Aching: Eup. purp., Hydrast., Zingib.
Dull: Hydrast.

In, and bladder, with dysurea: Eup. purp.

With frequent desire to urinate: Zingib.

Agonizing in a small spot over r. illium, with pain
in: Dios.

Burning drawing in: *Tereb.*

In, and in loins from cold, with hiccough
and burning in stomach: Coccin.

Constant: Canth.

Cramplike pressive, in, and in small of back:
Caust.

Darting, and chilliness, with painful urging which
dissappears when menses come: Kali i.

Digging tearing: *Berb.*

Dragging: pic. ac.

Dull aching: Hydrast.

And burning: Tereb.

Soreness and weakness, <r. side: Phyt.

In: Cup., Ferr., Ox. ac.

alt. with cloudiness as if drunk: Alum.

And in loins from cold. hiccough and burning
in stomach: Coccin.

As from knives: Arn.

If torn, and sticking: Mez.

From riding over rough roads, <from dancing:
Alum.

If desire to urinate is not complied with: Con.

Intense, <motion (Bry.) urine scanty, red and
hot, great pain on urinating, desire
constant day and night: Senec.

Pressive cramplike; and in small of back: Caust.

Tensive, and in loins, with feeling of stiffness, lameness and swelling in
back and lower limbs: Berb.

PAIN: In, Severe: Aloe.

    Violent, when lifting or blowing nose: Calc. p.

    <Sneezing, deep inhalation and lying down: Aeth.

    Sticking, violent, extending from: *Berb.*

    Tearing and soreness, esp. from exposure to wet: Rhus.

    Tensive in l.: Kali c.

PRESSING and drawing in r.: Aloe.

PRESSURE: *Berb.*, *Kali. c.*

    And tension: *Berb.*, Clem.

    Sensitive to: Phos., Tabac.

ROADS: See Pain in.

SENSITIVE: Acon.

    See Pressure.

SHOOTING in, small pulse and prostration: Kali bi.

SORE bruised sensation: Thuya.

SORENESS: *Apis.*, Berb.. Hep., Ipomea, Phyt., *Rhus.*

    And burning: Berb.

    Intense in l., pain, in back and along ureters, paroxysmal, with nausea and vomiting: Ipomea.

    Weakiness and dull pain, <r. side: Phyt.

    With urging to urinate, which is incessant: Hep., Merc. Corr.

STICKING and pain as if torn: Mez.

STITCHES: Berb., Cocc. c., Kali c., Lach., Phos. ac.

    To bladder: Berb., Cocc. c.

TENSION and heat: Natr. m.

TIRED feeling with inclination to rub parts and with frequent stretching backward of body: Mancinnella.

URINATE, pain in, and in bladder if desire to, is not complied with: Con.

URINATION: See Burning in.

VIOLENT sticking pain extending from: *Berb.*

WEAKNESS, soreness and dull pain in, <r. side: Phyt.

WET, pain and soreness esp. from exposure to: Rhus.

# SMALL OF BACK.

ACHE, tired, across, down thighs, during rest: Dulc.
ACHING: Acon., China, Cim., Dulc., Rhus.

> Dull: Aesc.
>
> In 1. side: Acon.
>
> Tensive, as from cramp or as if bruised and
> crushed, slighest motion causes crying

BED: See Pain Broken and Bruised.      [out: China.
BITING and gnawing: Canth.
BRUISED feeling and throbbing: Kali c.

> Feels: *Rhus.*
>
> Sensation in, and back and constant pain: Nux.
>
> See also aching and Pain bruised.

BURNING in: Verat.
COLD, lameness in, and neck from a: Dulc.
CORD: See Pain from.
CRAMP: See Aching tensive.
CRUSHED: See Pain tensive.
CUTTING and stitches to, from ossa pubes, wlth urging
>                    to urinate: Amm. m.
>
> Dragging and pain: Mag. c.
>
> Pressure as from a, edge across, while standing
>              or bending backward: Rhus.

DEBILITY: Phyt., Thuya.
DISLOCATED, Soreness as if, in sacro-illiac region:
DRAGGING, cutting and pain: Mag. c.      [Calc. p.
DRAWING: Con., Led., Plumb., Thuya.

> Stitches and severe pain with, through lumbar
>                  vertebrae: Con.
>
> See also Pain drawing.

EDGE: See Cutting pressure.
HEAD, vertigo 11 A. M., stitches on top of H. and pain in
>        S. of B., on rising from sitting: Caust.

HEAVINESS: Euphra.
HEAVY load, pain as from a: China.
HIPS: See Pain to.
KINK in, hindering deep inspiration: Acon.

KNEES: See Pain beaten.

Tired ache across, and in limbs esp. K.:Hydrast.

LAME: See Pain lame.

LAMENESS and stiffness: Kali c., RHUS.

In, and neck from a cold: Dulc.

LASSITUDE, painful: Col.

LOAD, pain as from a heavy: China.

MENSES: See Pain in and violent.

NECK, lameness in, and, from a cold: Dulc.

NUMB sensation: Acon.

PAIN; Above: Sulf.

Aching: Acon.. Aesc., Cim., Rhus.

Dull: Aesc.

In l. side: Acon.

Acute: Naja.

Beaten, as if: ARN., Dig., Mag. m. Nux, *Rhus*, Sil.

At night: fill.

And bruised, as if, in, and knees: Nux.

As if flesh had been, to pieces, on grasping it: Rhus.

Break, as if it would; Aloe, Bell., Cim., *Kali. c.*, Natr. m., Nux. *Plat.*

Broken, as if: Kali c., Natr. c., Nux m., Plat., Staph.

To pieces, as if everything were, in morning in bed: Staph.

Bruised: Amm. m., *Arn.*, China, Cina, Hep., Nux.

Aching: China. [Sulf.

Across, as if: Mag. m.

And beaten, as if; in, and in knees: Nux.

Crushed, slighest motion causes crying out: China.

Sharp pressive: Hep.

As if: Amm. m., *Arn.*, Bry., *China*, Nux.

On lying on back: Bry.

Not>by motion: Cina.

Or crushed, during rest or motion, could neither lie on back or side at night in bed: Amm.m.

With, feeling: *Arn.*, *China*, Cina, Colch., *Nux.*, RHUS.

When lying on: Bry., China.

Constant, and bruised sensation in, and back: Nux.

PAIN; Cord, from, down spermatic; after seminal emissions: Sarsap.

Cramplike; pressive: Caust.

Crushed: See bruised or and tensive.

Cutting dragging with: Mag. c.

Drawing: *Lach.*, Nitr. ac., Nitrum, Stram., Stron.c.,
*Thuya,* Val.

Extends down thighs: Cim., Dulc.. Nitr. ac.

During rest: Dulc.

Intolerable, extending upward and downward: Lach.

Tearing, violent, <pressure: Acon.

Dull aching: *Aesc.*, Cim.

Griping: Phyt.

Hips, to and, from r. side of pubes: Amm. m.

From: Fagop.

In: *Acon.*, AESC., Amm. m., Bry., Canth., Caust.,
*China.*, CIM., *Cina.*, Coccul., Colch.,
Con., Ferr., Hep.,Ign., KALI C., Lach.,
*Lyc.*, Mag., Mez., Naja, Natr. c., Nitr.
ac., NUX, Ox. ac., Petr., Phos., Phyt.,
*Puls.*, RHUS, Sec., *Sep.*, *Sil.*, Verat.

Liver and: Ferr.

Intolerable: China.

Knees: See beaten and.

Lame, as if and weak: Lach.

Like labor pains: Puls.

Load, as from a heavy: China.

Menses, in, and thighs at, B. <walking, thighs<
sitting: Mag. m.

See violent.

Paralytic: Coccul.

Peculiar, as from a stick lying across, being pressed
from without: Nux m.

Pressive: Canth., *Carbo. an.*, Caust.

Cramplike: Caust.

Very sensitive to every step: Carbo an.

Rising, on, from sitting: Ant. c., Arg. n., Caust., Sil.

With vertigo and stitches on
top of head: Caust.

Severe, when, from a seat, standing or walking (Ant. c.) : Agr. n.

Violent, when, from sitting, when walking:
Ant. c., Arg. n.

PAIN; Rising, when, from stooping: Phos.
 Rheumatic: Dulc., Rhus, *Verat.*
 Seat: See rising.
 Severe: Arg. n: Calc., *Carbo. v.*, China, Con.
  And stitches: Con.
  On rising from a seat: Ant. c., Arg. n. Sil.
         &gt;standing or walking:
            Arg. n.
 Sore: Natr. c.
 Spermatic cord, down, after emissions: Sarsap.
 Spine, on both sides of: Ox. ac.
 Sprain and stitches, as from a, &lt;rest, &gt; walking:
            Staph.
 Sprained: Caust., Oleum an., Petr., *Puls.*
  As if on motion: Puls,.
  Violent, as if: Caust., Oleum an., Petr.
 Sticking; violent: Calc. caust.
 Stiffness and: Lyc., Puls., Sil.
  Like a, when writing: Lauro.
  And, on rising from a seat: Sil.
 Stitches and: Con., Staph.
   Severe with drawing in lumbar verte-
       bræ: Con.
  See sprain.
 Stooping, as after long: *Dulc.*
 Tearing, drawing violent, &lt;pressure: Acon.
 Thighs: See menses.
 To hips from: Amm. m., Fagop.
 Violent: Ant. c., Arg. n., *Calc. caust.*, Hep., LYC.,
  *Mag. c.*, *Natr. c.*, Petr.
  In morning on rising; during menses: Lyc.
  Like clawing, drawing, sticking, working:
            Ign.
  Most, after walking: *Natr. c.*
 Walking difficult, which makes: Bry.
  Most violent, after: Natr. c.
  &lt;When: Hep.
 Weak and lame, as if: Lach.
 Weakness and: Sep.
  Much and: Sep.
 Writing, like a stiffness when: Lauro.
 Tensive, as if crushed or bruised: China, Rhus.
PAINFUL lassitude: Col.
  Also in lower extremities: Col.

PAINFUL stiffness, on motion: *Rhus.*
  Weariness: Clem.
PRESSIVE: See Pain pressive.
PRESSURE and tension: Clem., Lyc.
  As with a cutting edge, across, while standing and
    bending backward: Rhus.
PULSATIONS: Natr. c. and m.
    Violent: Natr. c.
SEAT: See Pain severe.
SEVERE bruised feeling and throbbing: Kali. c.
  See Pain severe.
SLEEP prevented by bruised sensation: *Rhus.*
SORENESS on touch: China, Nux.
SPRAIN, stitches and pain as from, $<$rest,$>$ walking:
           Staph.
STICKING: Calc. caust., *Merc.*, Verat., Zinc.
  See also also Pain sticking.
STIFFNESS: Carbo an., Kali c., *Rhus.*
    And lameness: *Calc. fluo.*, Kali c., *Rhus.*
     Pain: Lyc., Puls., *Rhus.*, Sil.
      On rising from a seat: Sil.
    Painful, on motion: *Rhus.*
STITCHES: Amm. m., Con., *Kali. c.*, Puls., Staph.,
             SULF.
   See Cutting and Drawing.
TEARING: Phos. ac.
   Across: Lyc.
TENSIVE: See Aching tensive.
THIGHS: See Pain drawing and menses.
THROBBING and bruised feeling: Kali c.
    Drawing in all limbs and: Lach.
TREMBLING: Cim.
VERTIGO: See Head.
WALKING: See Pain walking.
WEAK: Lach., Phos. ac., Psor., Sep.
   LIMBS esp. lower heavy, from sexual excesses:
           Phos. ac.
   See also Pain weak.
WEAKNESS: Ars., Cim., Nux, Psor., *Sep.*, Zinc.
  Much and pain. Sep.

# LUMBAR REGION.

ABSCESS: Calc. c.

ACHING: Cobalt., Convall., Helon., Naja, *Berb.*

And burning: Helon.

Dull, soreness, great prostration, pains>lying on back: Convall.

BURNING and aching: Helon.

Weakness: Bell.

CUTTING in: Thuya.

Rectum and anus with dull aching soreness in,>lying on back: Convall.

CRAMP and pressure in: Bell.

• In lumbo-sacral region and coccyx: Bell.

DEEP lancinations in: Ginseng.

DORSAL region: See Pain in.

HEAVY weight, sensation of, in lumbo-sacral region: Col.

See Pain heavy.

HIPS, weakness in, and, extending down lower extremities: Ox. ac.

See also Pain across.

KINK in, hindering deep inspiration: Acon.

KNEES, special affinity for lumbar region and: Berb.

LUMBAGO: *Aesc.*, Agar., *Aloe, Amm., Ant. t.,* Arn., Bell., BERB., Brom., BRY., CALC. FLUO., Canth., Cobalt., Col., Convall., *Ferr.,* KALI C., *Kali s., Kali p., Lyc.,* Magnol., Natr. m., NUX, *Ox. ac., Puls., Rhod.,* RHUS, Thuya, Val., Zinc.

After confinement: Kali c.

Failure of Bry.: LYC.

Rhus: CALC. FLUO.

All night, goes off on rising,>walking slowly about: Ferr.

Alt. with headache: Aloe, Brom.

Pain elsewhere: Magnol.

In thighs: Amm. c.

LUMBAGO; Alt. with piles: Aloe.

As if small of back were broken, pains shoot down backs of thighs (Cim.) : *Kali c.*

Back feels lame (*Rhus*), bruised (*Arn.*) as if broken (*Kali c.*), <nights in bed (*Ferr.*), inability to turn over, must sit up first, the longer he lies the worse he feels: *Nux.*

Extending to hips and thighs (*Cim.*, Kali c.), < rising from a chair (Kali p.) or stooping: Zinc.

From a strain: Arn., *Calc. fluo.*, Nux, *Rhus*, Ruta.

Great pain on attempting to rise (Kali p., Lyc., Puls.), >warmth (Ars., Mag. p.) and bending backward (Bell.) cold: RHUS.

Involving sacrum and hips (*Cim.*, Kali c.) <lying on back, >lying on side, but esp. >change of position (*Rhus*), pains laborlike (*Cim.*, *Puls.*), or sprained (*Arn.*) on motion: Puls.

Must sit up in bed to turn over. <A. M., early: Nux.

Pain aching, shooting, stitching, <sitting, after seminal emissions: Cobalt.

From back around body (Acon., Vib.) and down thighs (Cim., Kali c.). red and mucus sediment in urine: Berh.

In hips and thighs (Cim., Kali c.) and cramps in legs: Bell.

Intense in l. as if parts were strained (Rhus) < standing (Sulf.) and more so when sitting than when walking: Val.

Seems confined to small spots: Col.

Severe in lumbo, sacral region: Aesc.

Shifts about (Puls.) and is <from warmth (Rhus>) : Kali s

See also under head of Pain.

Pressive bruised pain in, and back early on rising, on turning trunk or while standing (Arg. n.), walking (Sabin., Zinc.): Thuya.

Severe, >pressing against something hard (Rhus) and lying on back (Puls.): Natr. m.

In loins and over kidneys, incessant desire to urinate (Eup. purp.), moaning, severe agonizing pains: Canth.

Sudden, sharp, lancinating pains, extending up and down back, rarely through to front. <3 A. M. (Caul., Verat.), can't remain in bed (Ferr.): Kali c.

LUMBAGO;

> Terrible pain extends over both kidneys down thighs
> (Cim., Nitr. ac.), extremely anxious to change
> position often (Rhus), but slightest movement
> causes one to shriek in agony, frequent desire
> to pass large quantities of urine (Ign.), but
> the extreme pain from motion causes one to
> desist, legs numb, weak and cold: Ox. ac.

Vertebrae feel as if rubbed against each other: Ant. t.

With retching on slightest effort to move: Ant. t.

<after rest: *Calc. fluo.*, *Kali p.*, RHUS.

> And just commencing to move (*Rhus*), esp.

> <on rising from sitting: *Kali p.*

> In rainy weather: Rhod.

<sitting: Cobalt,, *Rhus*, Zinc.

<walking in open air: Agar.

> While, feels as if one must lie down: *Kali c.*

PAIN; Aching: Cobalt., Convall., Helon., Naja.

> And burning: Helon.

> Dull: Convall.

> Shooting, stitching, < sitting, after emis-
> sions: Cobalt.

Across, passing to hips: Nux.

> Severe: Sulf.

Across: Kali bi., Kalm., *Nux*, *Sulf.*

Agonizing, severe: Canth.

Body, from back around. and down legs. red mucus
> sediment in urine: Berb.

Boring, with painful weariness: Bufo.

Burning, aching: Helon.

Constant, dull, heavy, in, and sacral region: Phyt.

Deep lancinating: Ginseng:

> Seated: Eup. perf.

Dorsal and, in, with constant sexual desire, severe
> erections etc.: Onos.

Drawing: Kali bi., Puls., Thuya.

> Extending to: Kali. bi.

> Tensive: *Puls.*, Thuya.

Dull, aching, soreness: Convall.

> Constant heavy, in, and sacral region: Phyt.

Fatigueing, as from standing long: Cina.

Great, on attempting to arise (Kali p., Lyc., Puls.)
> >warmth (Ars., Mag. p.) and bending back-
> ward (*Bell.*), <cold: Rhus.

PAIN, Heavy, at 5 P. M. extends to testicles: Abrot.

 Constant dull: Phyt.

In: Abrot., *Aesc.*, Agar., Aloe, Amm. c. and m.,
Ant. t., Aur., Bell, Berb., Brom., *Bry.*,
Calc. *lfluo.* and phos., Canth., Cina,
Cobalt., Col., Convall., *Ferr.*, Helon.,
KALI. C., Kali phos., and sulf., Led.,
*Lyc.*, Magnol., Natr. m., Nux, Onos.,
Ox. ac., Phyt., Plumb., Puls., Rhod.,
RHUS, Sulf., Thuya, Val., Zinc.

Hips and thighs and cramps in legs: Bell.

 (*Cim.*, Kali c.), extending to <rising
from a chair (Kali phos., Lyc., Puls.,
Rhus) or stooping (Aesc) : Zinc.

Intense in l. as if parts were strained (Rhus), <standing (Kali.bi., *Sulf.*, Verat.) and more
so when sitting (Cobalt.) than when
walking: Val.

Intolerable: Canth.

Labor like (Cim.) or sprained (Arn.) on motion: Puls.

Legs, in and, followed by violent trembling of L.:
 Bufo.

Paresis of lower extremities with coldness and pain
 in L. R.: Stry. phos.

Pressive bruised, early on rising, >on turning trunk
or while standing(Arg.n.), <walking
(Sabin.. Zinc.): Thuya.

 Or tensive: Berb.

 Tensive: Lyc.

Severe: Aesc., Amm. m., Sulf.

 Across: Sulf.

Sharp lancinating, sudden, extending up and down
back, rarely through to front, <3 A. M. (Caul.,
Verat.) can't remain in bed (Ferr.): *Kali.c.*

Shifts about (Puls.) and is>from warmth(Ars., Hep.,
Mag. p. Rhus): Kali s.

Shooting, aching, stitching, <sitting, after emissions:
 Cobalt.

Sitting, in, after: Led.

Spots, seems confined to small: Col.

Sprained, in as if: Hep.

 Or labor like, on motion: Puls.

Squeezed, in as if: Caust.

PAIN, Stitching: See shooting.

    Tearing: Canth.

    Tensive, drawing: Thuya.

        Or pressive: Berb.

        Pressive: Lyc.

    Terrible, extends over both kidneys, down thighs: See Lumbago terrible.

PAINFUL tension and pressure in, and renal region, extending down limbs: Berb.

    Soreness in: Bar. c.

    Weariness in, with boring pains: Bufo.

PRESSURE: See Painful.

SORENESS: See Aching dull, and Painful.

SPECIAL affinity for: *Berb.*, CALC. FLUO., RHUS.

    And knees: *Berb.*

STIFF, tendons of muscles so painfully, that thigh cannot be raised, it feels paralyzed: Aur.

TEARING: Nux.

TENDONS: See Stiff.

TESTICLES: See Pain heavy.

UTERUS, feeling as if, had descended and pressed upon rectum, causing cutting in rectum and anus, and dull aching soreness in, great prostration, pain>lying on back: Convall.

WEARINESS, painful, with boring pains: Bufo.

WEIGHT, sensation of a heavy, in: Col.

# SACRAL REGION.

ACHE, constant, in, and hips,<walking (Sabin., Thuya, Zinc.) and stooping forward: Aesc., Cim.

Violent, in S.-illiac or lumbar region, < walking (Sabin., Thuya, Zinc.) and stooping: Aesc.

ACHING, tensive as from a heavy load: China.

To, from above crest of illia, downward and inward: Berb.

BACK, feels as if B. would break, from pain across S.-illiac symphysis: Aesc.

See also Pain in.

BRUISED feeling: Col., Ginseng.

See also Pain bruised.

COCCYX, neuralgia of S. and C., esp. when riding in a carriage: Nux. m.

Painful drawing in, and C. and thighs while sitting: Thuya.

CONSTANT: See Ache and Pain dull.

Twitching motion: Agar.

DISLOCATED, soreness in S.-illiac region as if: Calc. p.

DRAWING: Hep., *Thuya*.

Painful, in, and coccyx and thighs while sitting: Thuya.

DULL: See Pain dull.

FATIGUE: See Pain pressive.

HEAVINESS and pressing on sitting,>motion: Aloe.

HEAVY load, tensive aching in as from a: China.

See also Pain heavy.

HIPS, constant ache in, and in H.,<walking and stooping forward: Aesc., Cim.

Shooting in, and H. and below knees: Sep.

Between H.: Sil.

See also Pain in.

NEURALGIA of, and coccyx, when riding in a carriage: Nux m.

PAIN; Ab. c., Abrot., *Aesc.*, Agar., Aloe, Calc. c., *Carbo an.*, Cham., *China, Cim.*, Ign., Lob. c., Merc., Nux m., *Puls., Sep.*, Tell., *Thuya*.

PAIN: Aching: *Aesc.*, China, Cim.

    Constant, in sacrum and hips, <walking and stooping forward: *Aesc.*, Cim.

    Tensive, in as from a heavy load: China.

    Violent, walking or stooping: Aesc.

Across, feels as if back would break: Aesc.

    Severe: Form.

And soreness: Sep.

Back: See in.

Blow or fall, as after a violent: Arn.

Break: See across.

Bruised: Cham., Hep.

    At articulations of, with pelvis: Hep.

    Very severe: Cham.

Constant: Aesc., Sep., Thuya.

    Aching, in, and hips, <walking and stooping forward: *Aesc.*

    Dull, across hips and: Aesc.

    Heavy, in, and abdomen, extends to thighs and legs: Sep.

Dull: See constant.

In: Abrot., Aloe, Ign., Thuya.

    And back and neck, feels as if wrenched, from overlifting: Calc.

    As after a violent blow or fall: Arn.

    During stool: *Carbo an.*

    Esp. at night: Cham.

    Extending through hips: SEP.

    Small of back and: Arn., Chel., Hep.

Fall or blow, violent, as after: Arn.

Heavy: See constant.

Hips, extends from S. R. through: Sep.

    And down thighs to knees: Sep.

Night, esp. at: Cham.

Pricking and shooting, with extreme tenderness: Lob. c.

Pressive as from fatigue in evening: Puls.

Severe, across: Form.

Shooting and pricking, with tenderness: Lob. c.

Soreness and: Sep.

Sticking: Colch.

    Violent: Natr. s.

Stool, during: *Carbo an.*

PAIN: Tensive, pressive: Acon.

    Thighs, to, down sciatic nerve, <pressing at stool (Carbo an.), coughing or laughing, lying on affected side (Bry., Kali i., Sil.), lying down at night (Berb.), <r. side: Tell.

        See hips.

    Violent: Agar.

    Wrenched, neck, back and, feel as if, with, from overlifting: Calc.

PAINFUL drawing in coccyx, thighs and, while sitting: Thuya.

PRESSING and heaviness while sitting, >motion: Aloe.

SHOOTING, violent, in, between hips: Sil.

SITTING: See Painful and Pressing.

SORENESS and pain: Sep.

    As if dislocated; or separated: Calc. p.

STITCHES, violent, <walking in open air: Agar.

STITCHING in, on breathing: Merc.

STOOL, pain in, during: Carbo an.

TENDERNESS, extreme, cannot bear slightest touch, pains shooting and pricking: Lob. c.

TENSIVE aching as from a heavy load: China.

WEAK feeling: Ab. c.

WRENCHED: See Pain wrenched.

# COCCYGEAL REGION.

ACHES and pains, pressing, tearing and shooting in: Calc.p.

ACHING, excessive, in neuralgia of: Fluo. ac.

BRUISED: See Pain bruised.

BLOW, sensation of numbness as from a; on sitting: Plat.

BURNING in when touched, from pain: Carbo an.

COXALGIA alt. with hæmoptoe: Led.

CRAMP. intense painful sensation of, in: Bell.

DRAGGING: See Pain dragging.

DRAWING: Thuya.

HÆMOPTOE alt. with coxalgia: Led.

ITCHING of os, must scratch until parts become raw and sore: Bov.

JERKING, tearing: Cic.

LANCINATING: See Pain lancinating.

MENSES: See Neuralgia.

MORBUS coxarius ($<$l. side): Stram.

NEURALGIA during menses: Cic.

Excessive aching: Fluo. ac.

Pulsating sticking when sitting, with pain between scapulæ: Paris.

$<$rising, must sit still: Lach.

$<$sitting, *Kali bi.*, Petr.

NUMBNESS, sensation of as from a blow while sitting: *Plat.*

PAIN: Calc. caust., Canth., *Carbo an.*, *Caust.*, Cic., Fluo. ac., *Kali bi.*, *Lach.*, Led., Petr., Paris., SIL., SULF.

Aching: Calc. p., Fluo. ac.

And aches, pressing, tearing, shooting, in: Calc. p.

Bruised: Carbo an., *Caust.*, SULF.

At night, on rising, as after a long carriage ride: *Sil.*

Dragging: *Carbo an.*

Violent in, and small of back: SULF.

PAIN; burning, which becomes a b. when touched: Carbo an.

    Dragging, bruised: *Carbo an.*

    Impeding every motion: Phos.

    Lancinating, shooting: Tarent. H.

                Tearing: Canth.

    Ride: See Pain bruised.

    Rising, bruised, on: Sil.

    Shooting, lancinating: Tarent. H

    Sticking, violent, in, and small of back: Calc. caust.

    Tearing, lancinating: Canth.

PAINFUL: Petr., SIL.

      On sitting: Petr.

      Sensation of cramp: Bell.

RAW: See Itching.

RIDE, bruised pain as after a long: Sil.

RISING, neuralgia<on: Lach.

    See also Pain bruised.

SENSATION of numbness, as from a blow, while sitting:
                                       Plat.

SITTING, neuralgia<on: Kali bi.

    Painful on: Petr.

    Pulsating, sticking when: Paris.

    Sense of numbness, as from a blow, while: Plat.

SORE, os itches, must scratch until: Bov.

STICKING and pulsating in, when sitting: Paris.

    See also Pain sticking.

STIFFNESS begins in, and goes up back: Ars.

TEARING jerking in: Cic.

# LOWER EXTREMITIES.

ABDOMEN: See Pain severe and Phlebitis.

ABDUCTORS mostly affected, in motory paresis: Lathyrus.

ACHING and soreness: *Eup. perf.*, Rhus.

> In legs, feel weak, esp. knees: Hydrast.

> See also Pain aching.

ACUTE: See Cramp and Drawing.

AGITATION and restlessness, great, with desire to cry: Tarent. H.

ANKLES: See Pain drawing and rheumatic.

BEATEN: See Pain beaten.

BLUE, cold, almost immobile: Ox. ac.

BLUENESS of l. from distended varices, with pressive pain during menses: Ambra.

BONES, aching as if in: Ruta.

> All sensitive to touch, esp. of: Mang. acet.

BRUISED and heavy, feel as if: Natr. c., Nitr. ac.

> Sensation: Sulf.

> See also Pain bruised.

CALVES, as far as, go to sleep, during day: Carbo an.

COITION, weakiness of, esp. above and below knees, after: Calc.

COLD, blue, almost immobile: Ox. ac.

> And feet icy in paralysis from: Dulc.

CRAMP and extremely acute pains: Plumb.

CRAWLING, tingling, tired, weak, restless: Calc. p.

CRURAL neuralgia (Pod., Sulf.), severe pain down crural nerve, <hot weather: Xanth.

CRY: See Agitation.

DEBILITY and weariness as from a long walk: Arg.n.

DRAWING, acute, as far as knees: Puls.

> See also Pain drawing.

DROPSY, painful, pits on pressure (Ars.), nights, A. M., profound melancholy: Aur.

DROWSINESS, much muscular soreness in, with weakness and: Myrica.

EMACIATED: Abrot.

FALTERING, staggering gait: Con.

FEET, Oedematous swelling of legs and: Acet. ac.

> Swelling from middle of legs down, with great heaviness of: Natr. m.

GAIT, staggering, faltering: Con.

> Limbs feel heavy like lead: Gels.

> Tottering, tremulous in motory paresis, abductors mostly affected. <wet weather, sensibility remains: Lathyrus.

GIVE way: Nayt. c.

HAMSTRINGS feel tight when walking: Amm. m.

HEAD, nodes on, and, immense: Still.

HEAVINESS: Alum., *Gels.*, Natr. c., PIC. AC., *Sulf.*, *Zinc.*

> And stiffness: Carbo v.

> Weakness: PIC. AC., Zinc.

> Of feet with swelling from middle of legs down: Natr. m.

> Painful: Sulf.

HEAVY and bruised, feel as if: Natr. c., Nitr. ac.

> Like a load, feel, staggering gait: Gels.

> When walking, staggers, (Gels.), must sit down: Alum.

HIP: See Pain rheumatic.

ICY cold in paralysis: Dulc.

IMMENSE nodes on head and legs: Still.

IMMOBILE, blue, cold, almost: Ox. ac.

ISCHIAS <r. side: Col.

JERKING in, and parts of lower portion of body: Natr. c.

KNEES, acute drawing as far as: Puls.

> Legs ache, feel weak, esp.: Hydrast.

> Weakness and trembling, esp. above and below: Colc.

> See also Pain rheumatic.

LEGS, nodes on head and, immense: Still.

> Oedematous swelling of feet and: Acet. ac.

> Phlebitis, soreness and swelling of, up to thighs and abdomen: Ham.

> Swelling from middle of, with great heaviness of feet: Natr. m.

LAMENESS and weakness in: Caust., Phos.

LEAD, feel heavy like, gait staggering (Con.): Gels.

MENSES: See Blueness.

MOTORY paresis, tremulous tottering gait, abductors
mostly affected, sensibility remains, <hot
weather: Lathyrus.

NEURALGIA, crural: Gnaph., Pod., Sulf., *Xanth.*

Severe pain down crural nerve, <hot
weather (Lath.): Xanth.

Sciatic: Acon.

NODES on head and, immense: Still.

NUMBNESS, feeling of, and great inclination of r. to go to
sleep: Kali c.

Feel as if wrapped tightly when sitting, also weakness and: *Plat.*

PAIN; Aching: Elat., *Eup. perf.*, Hydrast., Kali bi., Phyt.,
RHUS, Sulf.

And soreness: EUP. PERF.

As if in bones: Ruta.

Can rest but for a moment in any position:
RHUS.

Dull: Elat., *Sulf.*

And shooting in l. thigh, down sciatic
nerve to instep and out of toes:
*Elat.*

<lying down: Sulf.

Acute, extremely, and cramp: Plumb.

Beaten, as if, with much weakness: Sep.

Bone, as if in: Ruta.

Break, as if thigh would, on straightening out limb:
Val.

Broken, as if in marrow or as if bones were: Ruta.

Bruised: Zinc. ox.

Burning: Ars., Col., Iris.

>heat (Hep., Mag. p., Rhus): Ars.

Shooting down to foot, <motion: Iris.

Tearing extremely violent, <heat (Lyc.),
pressure (China) and flexing leg on
abdomen: Col.

<nights (Merc., Rhus): Ars., Salyc. ac.

With anguish and restlessness: Ars.

Crampy: Bell., Menyanth.

With stiffness in hip and ham: Bell.

Crazy almost from, it drives one out of bed (Acon.,
Ars., Ferr., Rhus, Verat.): and compels
one to walk the floor (Acon., Ferr.): Cham.

Descends anterior crural nerve (Xanth.) increasing in
intensity as it goes down: Pod.

PAIN; Descends posterior crural nerve: Gnaph.

    Dragging: Acon.

    Drawing: Merc., Mez., Nux, Plumb., Phyt.

        A. M. and P. M., in bed: *Sulf.*

        Pressive, in l., <ankle: Agar.

        Severe paralytic; extends from abdomen down into l.: Carbo v.

    Dull aching: Elat., *Sulf.*

        And shooting: See burning shooting.

        <on lying down: Sulf.

    Electric flashes, like, <3 A. M. (Caul.. Kali c.) must sit up and let leg hang out of bed, or walk the floor (Acon., Cham., Ferr.): Verat.

    Excruciating: Cham.

    Extends whole length of leg, <nights (Ars., Merc., Rhus.) and walking (Bry., Thuya), restless feet: Zinc.

    Formication: Arn., Lyc., Rhus.

    Great, extends to ramification of nerves and to toes: Gnaph.

    Intense, changing with numbness: Graph.

    Intermittent, sometimes throbbing: Ign.

        Periodical, remittent: Arg.n., Ars., Ferr., Ign., Natr. m.

    Irregular spells: Coff.

    Intolerable, while standing and esp. sitting (Mag.m.), >walking (FERR., RHUS): Val.

    Jerking, aching in hips, <hot weather(Lathy., Phos.; Calc. p., IGN., Rhus): Kali bi., Xanth.

    Lightninglike (*Mag. p.*, Thall., Zinc.), violent: PLUMB.

    Marrow, as if in or as if bones were broken: Ruta.

    Paralytic drawing, from abdomen to l.: Carbo v.

    Pressive: Phyt., Plumb.

    Pressive drawing, <ankle: Agar.

        During menses, in varices: Ambra.

    Rheumatic, in hips and thighs, <r. side and r. knee with stiffness and oedema of. ankles: Chel.

    Severe, down crural nerve: *Xanth.*

        Paralytic, drawing, from abdomen to l. leg: Carbo v.

    Shooting and dull aching in l. thigh, down sciatic nerve to instep and out of toes: Elat.

        In: Iris, Plumb.

PAIN; shooting like lightning downward: Acon.

    Tearing, burning, extremely violent, heat (Lyc.) pressure (Kali bi., Sil.), and flexing leg on abdomen: Col.

    Whole length of r., <A. M. (Aloe, Sulf.) or sitting up up (Mag. m.; Verat.>), >lying perfectly still (Bry.): Dios.

Stitching: Coff.

Tearing: Acon., Canst., Coff., Col., Kali i., Merc., Nux.

    Down limb, <at rest (Ars., Ferr., Verat.), >motion (Ferr., Verat.), <nights (Ars., Ferr., Merc.), >heat (Ars., Hep., Mag. p.; Lyc. <): RHUS.

    Shooting: See burning.

    Violent, down to foot: Phyt., Rhus.

Thigh: See break.

Throbbing, as though joints would burst: Ign.

    See intermittent.

Tingling: Acon.

With lame feeling: Arn., Led., Zinc. ox.

    Numbness: Acon., Rhus.

    Stiffness and weakness: Lyc.

<motion (Bry.) yet not>lying down: Ran. bulb.

<standing: Agar., Sulf.

\    L.: Agar.

Wrenched, as if hip joints were: Iris.

PAINFUL heaviness: Sulf.

PARALYZED, r. feels as if: Chel.

Seem as if: *Rhus.*

PARALYSIS, attacks of suffocation, internal heat, external cold, result of fright; anxiety: Cup.

From cold, limbs feel icy cold: Dulc.

See Motory.

PARALYTIC condition, after excesses, fever, or diphtheria Natr. m.

    See also Pain drawing.

PHLEBITIS after pregnancy: Lach.

    Soreness and swelling of leg up to thighs, extends to abdomen: Ham.

RESTLESSNESS: See Agitation.

RISING, stiffness and general soreness on: Eup. perf.

RHEUMATISM of: Cim., Led.

SCIATICA, Chronic: Ign.

>lying on affected side (Puls.; Sil., Tell.<): Bry.

>motion: *Eup. perf.*, Ferr., *Rhus*.

Can hardly put foot to ground, but no>while walking: Ferr., Rhus.

Caused by working in water,<limb hanging down (Verat.>),>elevating knee: Calc.

Chronic, intermittent,<winter (Rhus),>summer:Ign.

During pregnancy: Arn.

Either side: Acon., *Amm. m.*, Arn., Ars., Bry., Calc., *Col.*, *Gnaph.*, *Ign.*, Kali bi., Phyt., Plumb., Pod., *Rhus*, Ruta, Salyc. ac., *Val.*, Verat., *Xanth.*, Zinc.

Esp. in women (Puls.; Kali bi., males), pains< motion (Bry), yet not>lying down: Ran. bulb.

From injuries and contusions: Arn., *Ruta*.

Great pains, extending to ramifications of nerves, with feeling of numbness (numbness sometimes alt. with pain), pains extend to toes (Elat.): Gnaph.

If Rhus, Ruta or Sep. failed: Fluo. ac. (Calc. fluo.)
Bry. failed: Lyc.

Jerking aching pain in hip,<in hot weather (Lathy.; Calc. p., IGN., Rhus>): Kali bi.

Nerves, extremely sensitive as if uncovered, cannot bear to have anything touch affected parts (Arn., China, Led.): Bell.

Neuralgic: Acon.

Of females: Puls., Ran. bulb.
Males: Kali bi.

Pain, bruised, in thighs and legs, shooting and gnawing in shafts of bones, and violent tearing in joints: *Bell*.

Burning,<nights (Merc., Rhus): Ars., Salyc. ac.
Anguish,>heat: Ars.

Descends anterior crural nerve(Xanth.; Gnaph.,posterior) increasing in intensity as it goes down: Pod.

During paralysis or muscular atrophy,violent,lightninglike: Plumb.

Extending whole length of leg,<night(Merc.,Rhus) and walking (Bry.), feet restless: Zinc.

Extremely violent, tearing(Rhus), shooting (Elat.), burning(Ars.),<heat(Lyc.; Ars.>), pressure (Kali bi., Sil.) and flexing leg on abdomen: Col.

SCIATICA:

Pain from sacrum to thighs<pressing at stool, coughing, laughing, lying on affected side (Nux, Sil. Bry., Puls.>) lying down at night (Rhus); and on r. side: Tell.

In hips and thighs intolerable while standing and esp.<sitting (Mag. m.),>walking (Kali bi., Sulf., Verat., Thuya): Val.

Like electric flashes, < 3 A. M. (Caul., Kali c.) must sit up and let legs hang out of bed (must elevate knees: Calc.), or walk about (Ferr., Cham.) : Verat.

Seems to be in marrow of bones, as if bones were broken: Ruta.

Recurring in cold season (Calc. p., Rhus), with intense coldness and shivering,<nights (Ars., Ferr., Merc., Rhus), pains intermittent, sometimes throbbing: Ign.

Violent, of a boring character, lasting about an hour, always preceded by coldness, has to get up and walk about (Cham., Ferr.): Ign.

Tearing pains down to foot: *Rhus*, Phyt.

With painful contractions of hamstrings: Natr. m.

<nights (Merc.), anguish, burning pains > heat (Lyc. <) : Ars.

<sitting (Mag. m., Val.),>walking (Kali bi., Sulf., Thuya, Verat.), but entirely > lying down (Rhus, Tell. <) : Amm. m.

(L. S.) : L. side: Ars., CHAM., Elat., Eup. perf., *Iris*, *Kali bi.*, Led., Menyanth., PULS., Still., *Sulf.*, *Thuya.*

>lying on affected side (Puls.; Sil., Tell. <): Bry.

>motion: Eup. perf.

L. side,>walking (Amm. m., Sulf., Thuya, Verat.) and bending leg (Col.), <standing (Val.), sitting (Mag. m., Val.), lying (Rhus, Tell.), and on pressure (Col., Sil.) : Kali bi.

Hip to os calcis, almost crazy from pain, drives one out of bed and compels one to walk the floor (Ferr., Verat.): Cham.

In females (Ran. bulb.; Kali bi., males), cannot rest, yet motion < (Bry.): Puls.

Of a burning character (Ars.) shooting down to foot, much<motion (Bry., Puls.): Iris.

SCIATICA;

(L.S.) : L. side, parts cold, <evening until midnight(Puls.) and from warmth of bed (Merc.): Led.

Syphilitic: Still.

Thighs and legs spasmodically jerked upward (Sticta), pains generally > motion (Rhus): Menyanth.

Pains as if l. hip joint were wrenched: Iris.

Dull aching, <lying down (Kali bi., Rhus, Tell. ; Amm. m. >), affecting outer part of l. thigh: Sulf.

Shooting and dull aching in l. thigh, down sciatic nerve to instep and out of toes: Elat.

Tearing sticking along l. to tip of big toe: Ars.

(R.S.) ; R. side: Caust., COL., *Dios.*, Lach., RHUS, *Tell., Val.*

Pain from sacrum to thigh, < pressing at stool (Carbo an., Nux), coughing, laughing, lying on affected side (Nux, Sil.; Bry., Puls. >) and lying down at night (Kali bi., Rhus), and on r. side (Col., Rhus): Tell.

Shooting whole length of limb, r. side, <morning (Mangan.) or sitting up (Amm. m.; Kali bi., Rhus, Sulf., Tell. > ), >lying perfectly still (Bry.) : Dios.

Pains tear down limb, <rest and night, >motion and heat: Rhus.

Tearing pressure in middle of inside of leg, not <or>by motion or contact: Bell.

Sticking along limb to tip of big toe: Ars.

<after sleep: Lach.

<straightening out limb, feels as if thigh would break: Val.

SLEEP, whole r. leg feels numb and inclined to go to: See also Calves. [Kali c.

SORENESS, general, and stiffness, when rising to walk: Eup. perf., Rhus.

And aching: Eup. perf., Rhus.

See also Drowsiness.

STAGGERS: See Gait, Heavy.

STIFFNESS: See Heaviness, Soreness.

SWELLING: See Feet.

TEARING, sticking along limbs to tip of big toe: Ars.
<nights: Nit. ac.

THIGHS: See Twitching.

TIGHT: See Hamstrings, Wrapped.

TIRED: See Crawling.

TOTTERING: Lathyrus, Nux.

And unsteadiness: Nux.

TOUCH: See Bones.

TREMBLING: See Weakness.

TWITCHING and spasmodic adduction of thighs: Merc.

ULCERS, varicose, burn at night, discharge offensive, purple all around: Carbo v.

UNEASINESS, cannot lie still at night, has to change position constantly or walk about (Ferr.) to get relief: Ars., Rhus.

UNEASY<nights: Ars.

UNSTEADINESS and tottering: Nux.

WALK, seems as if one could, forever: Fluo. ac.

WEAKNESS: Ars., *Calc.*, *Coca*, *Merc.*, Phos., *Pic. ac.*, *Rhus*, Sil., *Zinc.*

And heaviness: Pic. ac., Zinc.

Trembling esp. above and below knees after coition: Calc.

Weariness esp. on ascending steps: Ars., Calc., Coca.

Great: Pic. ac., Rhus.

While walking in open air: *Rhus.*

Nights: Merc.

See also Wrapped up.

WEARINESS amounting to almost paralysis, <l.: Cann. i.

Of l., unusual at noon: Calc.

See also Debility.

WRAPPED up tightly, feel as if, when sitting, also numbness and weakness: Plat.

# HIPS.

ACHING as if paralyzed in, and thighs, they give out:
Verat.

See also Pain aching.

In gluteal region: Calc.

ANKLES: See Paralytic, Rheumatic.

ASLEEP, nates feel as if, stinging in small spots: Calc. p.

BACK and, feel as if falling apart>tight bandaging: Trill.

Violent bruised sensation in, and, painful on stooping: Sil.

See Pain.

BACKACHE affecting: Aesc.

BLOW or sprain: See Pain blow.

BOILS on nates: Phos. ac.

BONES: See Pain bruised.

BROKEN, painful as if: Phos.

BRUISED sensation in, thighs and neck from growth:
Phos. ac.

Violent in, and back, painful on stooping: Sil.

See Pain bruised, Shooting.

BURNING in: Mag. m., Nux.

See also Pain burning.

CARIES in, and heels, pus offensive: Calc. p.

Of r., l. leg atrophied and painful: Caps.

COLDNESS in gluteal region: Calc.

COUGHING: See Pain sticking.

CRAMP: Natr. m., Phos. ac.

CUTTING or sore aching in spleen extends to: Grind.

See Pain cutting.

DIGGING: See Pain digging.

DISEASE, acute pains extend to knee, pains<motion (Bry.,
Calc. p., Hep., Nux): Sil.

Effects of prolonged suppuration, with night sweats and diarrhœa: China.

DISLOCATED, joints pain as if: *Puls.*

DISLOCATION, pain as from: Lauro.

DRAWING: *Acon.*, *Carbo v.*, *Dulc.*, *Lyc.*, Rhus, Sep.,
Zinc.

In joint: Acon.

Extending down thighs, <walking: Carbo v.

L.: Acon., Rhus, Sep.

<on first moving: R$_{hus}$, Sep.

Rheumatic: Zinc.

Tearing from, to feet: Lyc.

In l.: Dulc.

See also Pain drawing.

DULL: See Pain dull.

FALLING: See Back.

FEET: See Coughing, Drawing, Rheumatic.

GNAWING: See Pain bruised.

GROWTH: See Bruised sensation.

HEELS: See Caries.

IMMOVABLE: See Joints.

INFLAMMATION: See Joints.

JERKING: See Joint, Pain jerking.

JOINT, almost immovable: Con.

Dislocated, pain as if: Puls.

Drawing in l.: Acon.

Extending down thighs, <walking: Carbo v.

Inflammation of, which is sore to pressure: Calc.

Pain, jerking: Mez.

Paralytic, in r., thigh and ankle, latter feels
as if sprained, unable to walk without
limping: Dros.

Pressive in both, on every step, with paralyzed
sensation in anterior muscles of
thigh: Rhus.

Tensive in r.: Nit. ac.

Rheumatic, in, and knee: Kali p.

Shooting: *Sulf.*

Violent: *Agar.*, Sulf.

<touch: Sulf.

Painful laxity of both, as if capsules were weak and
relaxed: Thuya.

Peg: See Tingling.

Shooting tearing, which pain as if bruised when
touched along tibia, <evening in bed: Ferr.

Rheumatism of, and knee: Led.

JOINT, stitches in r.: Natr. m.

    Suppuration: Calc. p. and s., *Hep.*, Sil.

    Tearing in, and knee, while sitting: Kali c.

        Violent: See Pain bruised.

    Tingling as if a peg were driven in: Bufo.

KNEE: See Disease, Joint, Pain, Sticking, Tearing.

LAMENESS of r.: Dios.

LANCINATING pains: Bufo.

LAXITY: See Painful.

LEG: See Caries, Pain bruised.

LIMPING: See Paralytic.

NATES painful as if suppurating: Phos.

    See Asleep, Boils, Sprain.

PAIN: Aching, in r.: Eup. perf.

    Acute: See Disease.

    Back, from, to small of: Fagop.

    Blow or sprain, as from a in, and thighs: Arn.

    Bruised: Bell., Form., Ginseng., Natr. m., Phos. ac.,
                        Sil., Zinc.

        ■   And tensive: Phos. ac.

    Bruised in bones of thighs and legs, shooting and
        gnawing in shafts of bones and violent
        tearing in joints: Bell.

    Burning, in bones: Eup. perf.

    Coughing, sticking tearing, from, to feet on: Caps.

    Cutting, violent, in r.: Ginseng.

    Digging, jerking, pinching: Cann. s.

    Dislocated, joints, as if: Puls.

    Dislocation, as from: Lauro.

    Drawing: Carbo v., Chel., Colch., Dulc., *Puls.*, Rhus,
                        Stram.

    Dull hard: Dios.

    From, to small of back: Fagop.

    In: Acon., *Arn.*, Cham., Colch., Dios., *Eup. perf.*,
        Fagop., Hell., Hep., Kali p., Nux, *Phos. ac.*,
        *Rhus*, Sep., SIL., Stram.

        And kidneys: Tarent.

            Knees: Rhus.

            Thighs extending to knees: *Sil.*

        Joint as if sprained: Hep.

            Violent: *Agar.*

                <touch: Sulf.

    Jerking: Mez., Nux.

PAIN: Jerking; in joint: Mez.

 Knee, in, and: Rhus.

  To from thighs and H.: Sep.

   R. H. while walking, cannot stand or bear any weight on limb: [Hydrast.

Lancinating: Bufo.

Leg: See bruised.

Muscles, in: Lyc.

Nates: See sudden.

Paralytic: Dros., Lyc.

  In r. joint, thigh and ankle. latter feels as if sprained, unable to walk without limping: Dros.

Pinching: Caust.

  See digging.

Pressive: RHUS.

  In both joints on every step, with paralyzed sensation in anterior muscles of thighs: Rhus.

  Tensive, in r. joint: Nit. ac.

Rheumatic: Carbo v., Chel., Form., Graph., Kali bi. and p., Kalm.

  Down to feet: Kalm.

  In, and knees: Kali p.

Rheumatic in, and thighs, < r. side and r. knee, oedema of ankles with stiffness: Chel.

Shooting: *Sulf.*

  In joint: *Sulf.*

Sticking: Calc. caust., Caps.

  In, and knee: Calc. caust.

  Tearing from, to feet, esp. on coughing: Caps.

Sprain, as from a: ARN., Euphorb., Phos.

 . See also blow and sudden.

Sprained, as if in joints: Hep. .

Sudden, on attempting to walk, as after a sprain, below r. nates: Mez.

Tearing: *Aesc.*, *Caps.*, Caust., Clem., Mag., Nit. ac.

  From, to feet: Caps., Sep.

   Knees: Canth.

  See sticking.

Tensive: Sulf.

  On walking: Sulf.

  See also bruised and pressive.

Violent, in joints, <touch: Sulf.

PAINFUL laxity in both joints as if capsules were too weak and relaxed: Thuya.

    Weariness: Bufo.

    See also Broken, Bruised, Nates.

PARALYZED: See Pressure, Walking.

PARALYTIC: See Pain paralytic.

PEG: See Tingling.

PRESSIVE: See Pain pressive.

PRESSURE: Pet.

    See also Inflammation.

RELAXED: See Weak.

RHEUMATISM in l. result of dry cold air: Acon.

    Of H. and ham, l.: Bell.

        Shoulder and knee: Carb. ac.

RHEUMATIC drawing: Zinc.

    Tension: Lyc.

    See also Pain rheumatic.

SHOOTING and tearing in joint, which pains as if bruised when touched along tibia, <evening in bed: Ferr.

SORE: See Joint.

SPRAIN: See Blow, Pain and Sudden.

SPRAINED: See Pain sprained and paralytic.

SPOTS: See Asleep.

STICKING: Nux.

    See also Pain sticking.

STIFFNESS: See Pain rheumatic.

STINGING: See Asleep.

STITCHES in r. joint: Natr. m.

STOOPING: See Bruised.

SUDDEN: See Pain Sudden.

SUPPURATION of joints: Hep.

    See also Disease, Nates.

TEARING in H. and knee joints, even while sitting: Kali c.

    See also Pain bruised and Shooting.

TENSIVE: See Pain tensive.

THIGHS and H. give out and ache as if paralyzed: Verat. a.

    See also Bruised, Drawing and Pain rheumatic.

THROBBING: Mag. m.

TINGLING as if a peg were driven in joint: Bufo.

TOUCHED: See Shooting.

'WALKING difficult, like from paralysis, first r. then l'.:
Verat. a.

WEAK, relaxed: See Painful.

—— ———

# THIGHS.

ACHING and soreness: Calc. p.

Dull, and shooting pain in l. to instep and out of toes:
Elat.

ANKLES: See Pain rheumatic and tearing.

BACK, pain in T. and small of B. at menses, T. <sitting,
B. <walking: Mag. m.

BEATEN, painful as if: Lauro.

See also Pain beaten.

BED: See Pain beaten.

BLOW: See Pain blow.

BONES, periostitis of, great sensitiveness to pressure and
burning pains extending into knee, parts
become erysipelatous and threaten to sup-
purate: Mez.

See also Pain bone, drawing and bruised, Sensation.

BORING: Mez.

BROKEN: See Pain broken.

BRUISED: See Pain bruised.

BURNING: See Bones, Pain burning.

CALVES: See Cramp and Drawing.

COLD and clammy: Calc., Merc.

COLIC extends to: Tereb.

CONDYLE: See Drawing.

CONSTANT: See Pain constant.

CRAMP: Sep.

At night: Carbo an.

In, calves and feet, with painless watery stools: Pod.

R.: *Sulf.*

Terrible: Digitalin.

CRAMPLIKE: See Pain cramplike.

CRAMPY: See Pain crampy.

DOGS: See Sensation.

DRAWING: *Col.*, Kali c., *Nux.*

DRAWING and tension in, and legs, evenings: *Puls.*

In external condyle of r. femur and esp. of knees on motion: *Col.*

Paralytic, (Nux) in whole T.: Kali c.

In muscles of, and calves, painful on walking: Nux.

Rheumatic: Zinc.

See also Pain drawing.

DROPS: See Water.

ERYSIPELATOUS: See Peritonitis.

EXOSTOSIS: Sil.

FEET, shooting to: Magnolia.

See Cramp.

FEMUR: See Drawing, Pain beaten.

FLUID: See Pain similar.

GNAWING: See Sensation.

GROIN: See Pain similar.

HEAVINESS and numbness: Aloe.

Stiffness: Bell., Pet.

Weakness: Lyc.

Weariness, paralytic: Sil., Stann.

Of, and knee joint: Sil.

HIP: See Blow, Pain crampy and rheumatic.

ILLIAC: See Pain similar.

INJECTION: See Pain similar.

INSTEP: See Aching.

JERKING tearing in anterior and outer portion of, only on touch, not by motion: China.

KNEE: See Drawing, Pain bruised, drawing, rheumatic, tearing.

KNIFE: See Pain similar.

LAMENESS in l.: Coccul.

LEGS: See Drawing, Weakness.

LIVER: See Pain liver.

MENSES: See Back.

NEURALGIC: See Pain Neuralgic.

NUMBNESS: See Heaviness, Weakness.

PAIN: Beaten, as if, in femur, while walking, sitting or lying, even mornings in bed, on waking: *Sil.*

Blow or sprain, as from, in, and hips: ARN.

Bones, from middle of, to knee, > waking (Rhus) < rest: Indigo.

See also drawing, bruised.

PAIN: Broken or bruised: Cham., Chel., Eup. perf.

 As if: Coccul., Eup. perf., Plat.

 Bruised: BELL., Mag. m., Mez., Nux, *Puls.*, Sep.,
              *Sul*

  In anterior muscles: Hep.

  Bones: *Puls.*, Bell., Eup. perf.

  T. and legs, shooting and gnawing in shafts of bones and tearing in joints: Bell.

 Burning. in bones, at night: Euphorb.

  See also Bones.

 Constant: Digitalin, Dulc.

 Cramplike: Crotal., Cyc., Plat.

  In posterior part of T. above popliteus: Cyc.

 Crampy (Gels.) tearing, in outer side of T. extending into hip: Val.

 Drawing: Carbo v., Cup., Natr. m., Phos. ac., Stram., Sulf.

  In bones as if periosteum had been scraped: China, *Phos. ac.*

  R. extends to knee: Natr. m.

 Rheumatic: Agar.

 Severe: Caul.

 Tearing: *Acon.*, Dulc., Natr. m., Nux.

  Or constant, at one time sticking, at another pinching, disappearing on walking, returning immediately on sitting: Dulc.

 Knee: See drawing, rheumatic.

 Lame, in, and upper arm: Coccul.

 Liver, into T. from: Cobalt.

 Neuralgic, in outer part: Phyt.

 Ovarian, extends to T. and returns at same hour each day: Cact.

 Paralytic: Chel., Cina.

 Pinching: See drawing.

 Rheumatic: Lach.

  Drawing: Agar.

  In r.: Kali bi.

  T. and hips, <r. and r. knee, oedema of ankles, with stiffness: Chel.

 Shooting: Form.

  And dull aching, in l., to instep and out of toes: Elat.

PAIN; Similar to injection of fluid or as if a fluid were forcing its way from l. illiac region, extending down l. groin to half way down front of l. T. and ends there in a sudden pain as from a jagged knife: Cocc. c.

  Sudden: See similar.

  Tearing: Aloe, Calc., Carbo v., Hep., Rhus.

  Above l. knee, extending down to near ankle: Indigo.

  Violent: Plumb.

PAINFUL and tense: Natr. m.

  As if beaten: Lauro.

  Posterior portion: Hep.

  Tension: Nux.

  Weariness: Bry., Calc.

  See also Drawing.

PARALYZED, seem, and bruised: Coccul.

PARALYTIC drawing: Kali c., Nux.

  Heaviness and weariness: Sil., Stann.

  Of, and knee joint: Sil.

PERIOSTEUM: See Pain drawing.

PERIOSTITIS: See Bones.

PRESSURE on l. toward posterior portion: Led.

REDNESS and swelling of inside of r.: Stram.

RHEUMATIC: See Drawing, Pain rheumatic.

SCRAPED: See Pain drawing.

SENSATION as if dogs were gnawing flesh and bones of T. and feet: Nit. ac.

SHOOTING down backs of: Kali c.

  To feet: Magnolia.

  See also Aching, Bones, Pain shooting.

SPRAIN: See blow.

STIFFNESS and heaviness: Bell., Pet.

  Weariness of anterior muscles, A. M. on beginning to walk: Calc.

  See Pain rheumatic.

. STICKING tearing: Dulc.

STITCHES from liver down: Cobalt.

SWOLLEN: See Redness.

TEARING: Bell., China, Lyc., Mez., Natr. c., Sep., Thuya, In middle: Indigo.                    [Zinc.

  Of r.: Lyc.

  See Jerking, Pain bruised, constant, drawing, tearing, Sticking.

TENSION: See Drawing.

TERRIBLE cramps: Digitalin.

TIGHTNESS: *Plat.*

TOE: See Aching.

TOUCH: See Jerking.

TREMBLING: See Weakness.

WALK: See Back, Pain beaten, drawing, Stiffness, Weariness.

WATER, sensation of drops of, trickling down front of: Acon.

WEAKNESS: Caust., Con., Hell., Lyc., Oleand., Verat.

And heaviness: Lvc.

Numbness and trembling: Con.

Of T. and legs: Oleand.

WEARINESS as after excessive effort: Rheum.

Excessive, with trembling of knees: Puls.

Of T. as after a long walk, A. M. on beginning to walk: Calc.

See also Painful, Paralytic, Stiffness.

# KNEES.

ACHE severely: Aesc.

 Tensive, from bends to heels: Rheum.

ACHING in outer part of l. while sitting, $<$ walkin
              Hydra

 Of patellæ, as if beaten loose: Bry.

ANKLES: See Pain rheumatic, Painful, Tearing.

BACK: See Weakness.

BANDAGED: See Paralyzed.

BEATEN, joints pain as if: Arn., Ars.

 Loose, patellæ ache as if: Bry.

 Or sore, pain as if: Arn., Led.

BEND, itching tetter in of: Kali ars. ·

 Tensive ache from, to heel: Rheum.

BONE: See Pain bone.

BORING and drawing: Col., Mez.

 See Pain boring.

BOUND, sensation as if too tightly: Sil.

 See Tremulous.

BROKEN: See Pain bone.

BRUISE: See Synovitis.

BRUISED feeling: Zinc.

 See Pain bruised.

BUBBLING: See Synovitis.

BURNING and dryness in patellae: Bufo.

CHRONIC synovitis: *Calc. fluo.*, China.

CLAWS: See Sensation.

COLD, intensely so in diabetes: Berb.

 Nose, hot K.: Ign.

COLDNESS: Col.

 In bed: Carbo v.

CONTINUOUS: See Pain continuous.

CONTRACTIVE pain: Ferr.

CRACKING: *Calc.*, *Caust.*, Chel., Coccul., Glon., Ig1
    *Led.*, Natr. s., *Puls.*, Sul.

CRACKING and creaking: Cham., Ign., *Led.*

    In joints with stiffness: Natr. s.

    On walking: Caust.

CREAKING: See Cracking.

CRAMP: Hep.

    In hollows: Calc.

CRAMPLIKE drawing: Oleand.

    See also Pain cramplike.

CUTTING shoots in external muscles above r., only on sitting: Bell.

DIABETES, intensely cold in: Berb.

DIGGING: See Patellæ violent.

DRAGGED down, pateilæ feel: Cann. i.

DRAWING and boring: *Col.*, Mez.

    Tearing, violent, through, and tibia, esp. evenings: *Sulf.*

    Tension: Cham.

    Cramplike: Oleand.

    Painful, with weakness, when standing or walking which is very difficult, K. give way: Cup.

    Rheumatic: Iod.

    Stitches in r., < motion: Staph.

    See also Pain drawing.

DROPS: See Synovitis.

DRYNESS and burning in patellae: Bufo.

DULL pain: Clem.

EFFUSION: See Synovitis.

EXUDATION: See Synovitis.

FALL: See Weak.

FEET, stiffness of, and: Ars., *Rhus.*

    Alt. with tearing pains: Ars.

    See also Tremulous.

FIRMNESS, joints have none: Arn.

GIVE way, excessive weakness: Merc.

    See also Drawing painful.

GOUT: Calc.

GOUTLIKE tension: Phos.

GOUTY pains: Crotal., Pet.

HANDS: See Tendons.

HARD: See Swelling.

HEEL, tensive aching from bend of K. to: Rheum.

HIPS: See Pain rheumatic, sticking.

HOLLOWS, cramp in: Calc.

 Hard swelling in: Mag. c.

 Painful as from stiffness: Nit. ac.

  On motion: Natr. c.

 Stiffness of: Sulf.

  And tension: Nux.

 Tendons seem too short: Natr. m., Nux.

 Tension: Dig., Nux, Sulf., Verat.

  On stepping as if too short: Sulf.

 See also Pain, Sensation, Stiffness.

HOT swelling of r.: China.

 Nose cold: Ign.

HOUSEMAID'S: Iod., Sticta.

HYGROMA patelae: Arn.

ITCHING tetter in bends: Kali ars.

JERKING pain: China.

JOINTS have no firmness: Arn.

K. caps ache as if beaten loose: Bry.

KNIFELIKE pain in joints: Acon.

KNOCK together: Agar., Bry., Chel.

  And totter while walking: Bry.

KNOCKING under and tottering of: Nux.

LAMENESS and painfulness of l.: Crotal., Dios.

LEG, stiffness of, L. and r. big toe: Atrop.

 See Stiffness, Weak.

LOSS of power: Bry.

NEURALGIA under, >warm wraps: Atrop.

NOSE cold K. hot: Ign.

NUMBNESS: See Synovitis, Tremulous.

PAIN; Aching: Aesc., Bry., Hydrast., Rheum.

 And trembling: Chel.

 Beaten, as if in joints: Arn., Ars.

  Or sore, as if: Arn., Led.

 Bone, in, just below K., as if it had been broken and were not perfectly firm, while stepping upon it: Verat. a.

 Boring: *Canth.*, Sep.

  Nightly in synovitis (q. v.): Iod., Merc.

  <nights (Iod.), K. swollen (Apis, Bry., Puls.) in rheumatism: Kali c.

 Broken: See bone.

 Bruised: Acon., Cic., *Graph.*, Lach., Natr. c.

PAIN; Bruised and sprained, as if: Ars.

        At night: *Graph.*

    Continuous: Colch., *Col.*

            In 1. joint on motion: Col.

    Contractive: Ferr.

    Cramplike: Pet.

    Dislocated: Bufo.

    Drawing: Acon., *Caust.*, *Col.*, *Cup.*, Natr. m., PULS., Rhus.

        In bends: Cyc.

        Tearing: *Puls.*

        While sitting: Natr. m.

  Dull: Clem.

  Felt most on first moving, in the morning, in synovitis: Rhus.

    Fatigued: Verat.

    Gouty: Crot. h., Pet.

  In hollows: Natr. c., Nit. ac.

   L. as if bruised and sprained: Ars.

  Intolerable, with swelling: Lach.

  Jerking: China.

  Knifelike in joints: Acon.

  Neuralgic: *Atrop.*, Bell.

  Rheumatic: Bry., Cim., Clem., Phyt., Puls., Rhus.

        In r., hips and thighs, <r., ankles oedematous and stiff: Chel.

  Severe, with rheumatism: Ferr. p.

  Sharp in 1.: Caul.

  Sore: See beaten.

  Sprain, as from a: Lach., Lyc., Nit. ac.

        In r.: Lach.

  Sticking in, and hips: Calc. caust.

  Stiffness as from a, on rising from a seat: Sulf.

  Stiff: Oleand.

  Stinging, as from a bruise in synovitis: Apis.

  Tearing: Acon., Ars., *Puls.*

        Alts. with stiffness of, and feet: Ars.

        Drawing: Puls.

           In joints: Acon.

  Tensive: *Bry.*, Caps.

  Under patella: Rhus.

  Violent in both legs, cannot walk, K. stiff: Calotropis.

        And pressure: Natr. s.

PAINFUL: Mag. c.

    As from stiffness in hollows: Nit. ac.

    Hollows, on motion: Natr. c.

    Stiffness: Bry., Dros.

            Of, and ankles: Dros.

            Tensive: Bry.

    Swelling: *Nux.*

    See also Drawing.

PAINLESS swelling: Puls.

PALMS; See Tendons.

PARALYZED or bandaged, feel as if, patient is scarcely
            able to walk: Anac.

PATÉLLAE, burning and dryness in: Bufo.

    Dragged down, feel: Cann. i.

    Hygroma: Arn.

    Pains under: Rhus.

    Severe pressure below: Chel.

    Snap sideways: Cann. s.

    Violent tearing, raging, digging up under: Arg. n.

PRESSURE, severe, below patellae: Chel.

    See Pain violent, Severe, Weakness.

RHEUMATIC drawing: Iod.

    See also Pain rheumatic.

RHEUMATISM: Apis, Bry., Ferr., Kali c., Puls., Rhus,
                     Sticta, Sul.

    Esp. r., >motion, pains boring<nights, K. swollen:
                     Kali c.

    Of shoulder and: Kreos.; R. side: Apoc. and.

        Hip and, 1. side: Verat. v.

    With severe pains: Ferr. p.

SENSATION as if articular surfaces were separated:
                     Cham.

        Bound too tightly: Sil.

        Claws were clasping: *Cann. i.*

        As if hollows of, were too short, when rising
            from a seat: Nux.

    In hollows as if tendons were too short: Natr. m.,
                     Nux.

    Of great fatigue: Merc.

    See also Synovitis, Tremulous.

SENSITIVENESS: See Synovitis.

SEVERE pressure below patellae: Chel.

    See also Pain severe.

SHOOTS: See Cutting.

SIDE: See Weak.

SEAT: See Pain, Stiffness.

SINK down from weakness: Coccul.

    See also Weak.

SITTING: See Aching, Cutting, Pain drawing, Tearing.

SORE: See Pain beaten.

SPRAIN: See Pain sprain.

STANDING: See Stiffness, Weakness.

STICKING: Natr. m., *Sulf.*

    And tearing in r., extending to feet: Sulf.

    In l.: Natr. m.

    See also Pain sticking, Swelling.

STIFFNESS: Ars., Caust., Bry., Nux, Rhus, Sulf.

    And tension in hollows esp. after standing: Nux.

        Swelling, cannot walk, with violent pains in both legs: Calotropis.

    In hollows: Sulf.

    Joints crack: Natr. s.

    Of, and feet: *Rhus*; Alt. with tearing pains: Ars.

        L., leg and r. big toe: Atrop.

    Painful in hollows as from: Nit. ac.

        Of, and ankles: Dros.

        Tensive: Bry.

    See also Pain rheumatic.

STITCHES: Bry., Nit. ac., Pet., Staph.

    Drawing in r., <motion: Staph.

    When walking: Bry.

SWELLING: Apis, Bry., Calc., Calotrop., Cist., Hep., Led., Lyc., Nux, Puls.

    And tensive sticking in, when walking: Led.

    Hot, of r.: China.

    Painful: Nux.

    Painless: *Puls.*

    White, sluggish: Calc., Cist.

SYNOVITIS: Apis, Bell., Calc. fluo., China, Rhus, Sulf.

    Chronic: Calc. fluo., China.

    Considerable exudation: Bry., Led., Sulf.

    Fistulous openings discharging bloody serum, nightly, boring pains: Iod.

    From sprains: Ruta.

SYNOVITIS, K. swollen, shiny, stinging pains, from a bruise: Apis.

Of, joint, with sensation of bubbling as from drops of water: Bell.

L., pain felt most on first moving in morning: *Rhus.*

With effusion (Bry.), great sensitiveness, trembling and numbness of extremities on attempting to walk: Led.

TEARING: Acon., Arn., Calc., Indigo, *Kali c.*, Lyc., Puls, RHUS, *Sil.*, Sulf., Thuya.

Frequent: Kali c.

In, and ankles at rest: RHUS.

Bends: Val.

Pressure: Led.

Sticking in r., extending to feet: Sulf.

While sitting goes off on motion: Sil.

See also Drawing, Pain tearing, Weakness.

TENDONS under, and in palms of hands, contracted: Canst.

See also Sensation.

TENSION in hollows: Dig., *Sulf.*, Verat.

On stepping, as if too short: Sulf.

Bends: Lach.

See also Stiffness.

TENSIVE ache from bends of, to heels: Rheum.

Stiffness, painful: Bry.

See also Pain tensive, Swelling.

TETTER, itching, in bends: Kali ars.

THROBBING: Merc.

THIGHS: See Pain Rheumatic.

TIBIA: See Drawing.

TIGHTLY, sensation as if bound to: *Sil.*

See Tremulous.

TOE, stiffness of l., and leg and r. big: Atrop.

TOO SHORT, tension in hollows on stepping, as if: Sulf.

See also Tremulous.

TOTTER and knock together when walking: Bry.

Under: Nux.

See also Weak.

TREMBLING and pain: Chel.

See also Synovitis.

TREMULOUS numb sensation as if too tightly bound, extends to feet: Plat.

UNSTEADINESS of: Acon.

WALK: See Paralyzed, Stiffness, Synovitis.

WALKING, cracking on: Caust.

> K. knock together and totter when: Bry.
>
> Stitches when: Bry.
>
> Swelling and tensive sticking when: Led.
>
> See also Drawing, Weak, Weakness.

WEAK, legs feel, esp. K.: Dig., Dios., Hydrast.

> Mornings: Dios.
>
> Threaten to sink, totter when walking and threaten to fall to one side: Coccul.

WEAKNESS: Ars., Dig., Dios., Led., Merc., Sil.

> Excessive, and giving way: Merc.
>
> Of joints and tearing pressure when walking, extending downward: Led.
>
> See also Drawing.

WEARINESS: Calc., Lyc.

WHITE swelling: Calc., Cist.

> Sluggish: Calc.

# LEGS.

ABDOMEN, drawn up to: Arg. m.

ACHE dreadfully: Agar.

>Severely: Aesc.

AIR, L. and feet feel as if floating in (Apis: body): Sticta.

ANASARCA (Ars., Lyc.) <toward night (Merc.) with anæmia and general sensitiveness of surface of body to slightest touch: China.

ANKLES: See Calf cramp.

ASLEEP, seem as if on rising from sitting: Puls.

BEATEN: See Pain beaten.

BLUENESS: See Veins.

BONES, drawing and tearing in: Kali c.

>Nodes on shin: Cinnab.

>See also Tibia.

BRUISED sensation: Cham., Col.

>Through: Cic.

>See also Pain bruised.

BURNING: Agar.

>See also Pain burning, Ulcers.

CALVES: Beaten, feel as if: *Eup. perf.*

>Boring: Mez.

>Cramp: Acon., Ambra, *Anac.*, ARS., *Calc. c.* and *p.*, Camph., *Caust.*, CUP., *Graph.*, Hep., Jatropha, Lyc., Phos., Plumb., *Pod.*, *Rhus.*, SEC., SULF., Merc. corr., *Verat. a.*

>>Day and night: Graph.

>>From ankle to: Cup.

>>In, and hollows of knees on stretching out leg: Calc.

>>Legs: Ambra, SULF.

>>Even when walking: *Anac.*, Calc., Sulf.

>>>They are painful as if too short: Sulf.

CALVES: Cramp in thighs and feet with painless stools: Pod.

On stretching out legs, at night: Sulf.

Violent, nights: Ambra, Calc., Sulf.

When walking: *Anac.*, Calc. p., Sulf.

'Or rising from a seat>lying down: Anac.

Debility: Arg. nit.

See also Rigidity.

Drawing and pressure: Nitrum.

Paralytic: Nux.

See also Pain biting.

Feet: See Cramp.

Hollows of knee: See Cramp.

Jerking, spasmodic: Opi.

Knee: See Cramp.

Pain: Colch.

Biting, sticking, tingling: Berb.

Bruised, paralytic: Mag. m.

Sticking: See Biting.

Tearing, in outer side: Val.

Tensive: Natr. m., Nux.

While walking: Natr. m.

Tingling: See biting.

Twinging, in outer side when sitting: Val.

Violent: Sec.

Painful: See Cramp.

Pressure: Cic.

Tension: *Carbo an.*, Puls.

Painless stools with cramps in C.: Pod.

Paralytic drawing: Nux.

See also Pain bruised.

Rigidity with debility and weariness as after a long walk: Arg. nit.

Rising: See Cramp.

Seat: See Cramp.

Severe tearing in tendons beneath r. C.: Caust.

Sitting: See Pain twinging.

Soreness: Aesc.

Spasmodic jerking: Opi.

Sticking: See Pain biting.

Stretching: See Cramp.

CALVES; Swelling: Dulc.
>    Tearing: *Caust.*, Mez., Natr. c.
>        See also Pain tearing.
>    Tendons: See Severe.
>    Tension: Natr. m.
>    Too short, feel as if on walking: Sil.
>        See also Cramp.
>    Thighs: See Cramp.
>    Violent cramp in C. at night: Ambra, Calc., Sulf.
>    Walking: See Cramp, Pain tensive.
>    Weariness: See Rigidity.
COLD, to knees: Calc., Sep., *Sil.*
COLIC pains extend to: Kali c.
CORDS were tied about, sensation as if: China.
CRAMPS: Ars., *Carbo an.*, Cham., Colch., Col., *Cup.*,
>        Jatropha, Pod., *Sec.*
>    Ankles to calf: Cup.
>    In forepart near tibia, on walking: Carbo an.
>    Occasionally, and in feet: Sec.
>    See also drawing.
CRAMPLIKE: See Pain cramplike.
CRAWLING, severe: Carbo v.
>    See also Tremulous.
CROSSED, cannot sleep unless: Rhod.
DEBILITY felt mostly in: Arg. nit.
DRAWING: Graph., Led.
>    And pains: Acon., Lyc.
>        Tearing in bones: *Kali c.*, Nit. ac.
>        Tension: *Puls.*
>    Heaviness and numbness.: Bufo.
>    Painful, cramps in calves, feet swell: Ferr. ac.
>        In tibia: Anac., Merc.
>  .    Pressure, jumping: Agar.
>    Rheumatic, in both: Carbo v., Graph., Mez.
>    Spasmodic: Nux.
>    See also Pain drawing.
DRAWN, up to abdomen: Arg. nit.
FATIGUE and weakness: Tarent.
FEEL as if they would burst on letting them hang down:
>                                    Vipera t.
FEET, swelling of l. L. and: Lach.
>    See also Drawing, Tearing.

FIDGETY: Tarent. h., Zizia.

GANGRENOUS death: Carbo v., *Sec.*

    See also Tibia.

GARTERS: See Sensation.

FORMICATION: Sec.

HEAD: See Nodes.

HEAVINESS: Con., Lyc., *Natr. m.*, Puls., Tarent.

    And paralytic weakness: Bell.

        Stiffness: Carbo v., Chel.

        Tension: Kali bi.

        Weariness as after a long walk: Rhus.

    During day: Puls.

    Feeling of: Agar.

    See also Drawing.

HIVES, small elevations like, on scratching: Spig.

JERKING and tearing, deep: Ars.

JUMPING drawing pressure: Agar.

MENSES: See Veins.

NODES on head and, immense: Still.

        Shin bones: Cinnab.

NUMB, easily get: Bufo.

NUMBNESS: Kali c., Plat.

    See also Drawing, Tremulous.

PAIN: Aching: Puls., *Rhus*, Sep.

    And drawing: Acon., Lyc.

    Beaten: See violent.

    Bruised: Carbo v.

        As if: Bell., Calc., Dios.

        And soreness to touch, in periostitis of tibia:
               Phos.

    Burning: Agar.

        <nights: See Tibia.

    Colic, extends to: Kali c.

    Cramplike: Hep.

    Deep pressive: Agar., Nitrum.

    Down to feet: Kalm.

    Drawing, in tibia: Merc.

    In: Bufo, Dios., Glon., Mez., Plumb., Psor., Rhus.

    Increasing when standing: Agar.

    Pressing in r. tibia: Mez.

    Pressive: See Veins.

    Pricking: See Ulcers, Veins.

PAIN; Rheumatic: Asclep., Kalm., Merc.

    Severe, esp. at night: Plumb.

    Sharp: Iod.

    Stinging: See Ulcers, Veins.

    Tearing, in backs of both, esp. in tendo-Achilles and calf, <standing or walking: Ign.

    Tearing in muscles: Staph.

    Violent, in tibia, as if beaten or as if periosteum were torn off: Mez.

PAINFUL: Ars.

    Drawing, cramps in calves, feet swell: Ferr. ac.

        In tibia: Anac., Merc.

    Varices, during pregnancy: Mill.

    Weakness: Aloe.

    Weariness: Calc., Caust.

PARALYTIC heaviness and weakness: Bell.

                  Feeling of: Coccul.

PERIOSTEUM: See Pain violent.

PERIOSTITIS: See Tibia.

PRESSING pain in r. tibia: Mez.

PRESSIVE: See Veins.

PULLED by, sensation as if being: Agar.

RHEUMATIC drawing in both: Carbo v., Mez.

    'See also Pain rheumatic.

RIGIDITY: Plat.

    See also Tremulous.

SENSATION as if being pulled by: Agar.

        Garters were too tighgt and, would go to sleep: China.

    See also Tremulous.

SEVERE crawlings: Carbo v.

    See also Pain severe.

SHAKE: Lyc.

SHARP pains: Iod.

SITTING, seem as if asleep on rising from: Puls.

    See also Tremulous.

SLEEP, cannot, unless L. are crossed: Rhod.

    L. and feet go to, as far as calves, during day: Carbo an.

SORENESS: See Tibia, Veins.

SPASMODIC drawing: Nux.

STANDING, pains increase on: Agar.

STIFFNESS and heaviness: Carbo v., Chel.

STINGING: See Veins.

SWELLING: Acet. ac., Calc., Chel., Clem., Cup., Iod., Kreos., Lyc., Natr. m.. Plumb.. Stram.

    Deep red, extending down: Lach.

        Like bruises: Bufo.

    Of, and foot: Lach.

    See also Drawing, Tibia.

TEARING: *Bell.*, Calc., Lyc., Natr. c., *Zinc.*

    And drawing in bones: Kali c., Nit. ac.

        Jerking, deep: Ars.

    Downward in tibia to back of foot: Zinc.

    In r. tibia: Kali bi.

    See also Pain tearing.

TENSION and drawing: Puls.

TIBIA: Cramp in fore part of, near T. on walking: Carbo an.

    Gangrenous periostitis, with bruised pain and soreness to touch: Phos.

    Painful drawing in: Anac., Merc.

    Periostitis of l. and of long bones, with burning pain <nights (Ars.), with soreness and swelling of periosteum: Mez.

    Tearing downward in T. to back of foot: Zinc.

        In r.: Kali bi.

    See also Pain drawing.

TOO tight: See Sensation.

TREMBLING: Cic., Lyc.

    And weakness: Bell., Calc.

    Visible, of one L.: Cic.

    Violent: Cic.

TREMULOUS crawling uneasiness in, while sitting, a sensation of numbness and rigidity, esp. <evenings: Plat.

TWITCHING: Merc.

UNEASINESS: Hep., Plat.

    See also Tremulous.

ULCERS, foul: Brom.

    Varicose, burn nights, discharge offensive, purple all around: Carbo v.

        Pains pricking and stinging, veins sore, but not the Arn. soreness: Ham.

VEINS, varicose, painful during pregnancy: Mill.

# LEGS.

VEINS; Varicose, distended, blueness of L. from, with
pressive pains during menses:
Ambra.

Sallow skin, orange urine, yellow stools,
etc.: Card. m.

See also Ulcers.

WALKING: See Tibia, Weariness.

WEAKNESS: Arg. nit., Aloe, Clem., Coccul., Dig., Merc.,
Oleand., Pic. ac.

And fatigue: Tarent.

Trembling: Bell., Calc.

Feeling of: Agar.

Painful: Aloe.

Paralytic, and heaviness: Bell.

WEARINESS: Crot. h., Dig., Hep.

And heaviness as after a long walk: *Rhus*.

Weakness, great: Cham.

Painful: Calc., Caust.

---

# ANKLES.

ACHE: Sep.

ACUTE: See Pain acute.

AGONIZING: See Pain agonizing.

BONES, pressure in, of, and lower portion of l. leg, in A.
M.: Led.

BORING: Mez.

BRUISED: See Pain bruised.

BURNING, drawing and sticking: Kreos.

CHILDREN: See Walk.

CONTRACTIVE pain: Ferr.

CRACKING in, joint, while walking: Nit. ac.

With pains: Hep.

CRAMP from, to calf: Cup.

DIARRHOEA, copious with rheumatic pains in: Propy.

DISLOCATED or sprained easily: Natr. c.

DRAWING: Indigo.

And pressure: Natr. s., Nitrum.

Burning and sticking through: Kreos.

See also Pain drawing.

FEET, itching intense on top of F. and A.: Led.

    Bend under when stepping on them: Natr. c,

    Heaviness of F., great, and esp. A.: Sulf.

    Turn easily, child walks on A.: Brucea.

    See also Pain bruised.

GOUT: See Inflammation, Pain gouty.

HEAVINESS, painful: Cup.

    See also feet.

INFLAMMATION, rose colored, gouty of joints: Phos.

ITCHING, intense on top of feet and A.: Led.

LAME and painful: Dios.

LAMENESS, general, after sprains, esp. of A. and wrists:
                        Ruta.

MALLEOLI, stiffness about: Sulf.

PAIN: Acute: Cyc.

    Agonizing, severe, in, wrists fingers and toes: Act.
                        spic.

    Bruised, as if, sudden, in outer malleolus of r. foot,
                pain felt more when standing,
                than when walking: Val.

    Bruised: Natr. m.

    Contractive: Ferr.

    Drawing: Caul.

        Pressive: Agar.

    Gnawing: Graph.

    Gouty: Pet.

    Intolerable: Led.

    Rheumatic, sharp: Form.

        With copious diarrhoea: Propy.

    Severe: Phyt.

    Severe: See agonizing.

    Sharp rheumatic: Form.

    Shooting, in rheumatism: Ferr. p.

    Sprain, as from a: *Phos.*, SULF.

            In l. on standing or walking: *Sulf.*

    Sprained, as if: Chel., Dig., *Phos.*

        On walking: Phos.

PAINFUL and lame: Dios.

    Heaviness: Cup.

    When touched: Ars., China., Lach.

PARALYTIC tearing: Dros.

PRESSING: Indigo.

PRESSURE: Clem., Hell.

    See also Bones.

PUFFINESS about instep: Ruta.

RENDING, shooting, tearing: Calc. p.

RHEUMATIC: See Pain rheumatic.

RHEUMATISM of, and wrists, with puffy swelling: Rut

    Of joints: Merc.

    Pains shooting: Ferr. p.

SENSITIVE: See Ulcers.

SEVERE: See Pain agonizing, severe.

SHARP: See Pain sharp.

SHOOTING: See Rheumatism, Rending.

SPRAIN or dislocate easily: Natr. c.

SPRAINS: See Lameness, Pain sprained, Stitches.

STANDING: See Pain bruised, sprained.

STICKING, drawing, burning: Kreos.

STIFFNESS: *Caust.*, Dros., Graph., Pet., *Sulf.*

    About malleoli: *Sulf.*

STITCHES as if sprained: Lyc.

SUDDEN: See Pain bruised.

SWELLING: Ferr., Led., *Ruta.*

    About joints: Merc.

    Puffy, with rheumatism: Ruta.

TEARING: Berb., Cham., *Kali c.*, *Rhus.*

    Rending, shooting: Calc. p.

TENSION on motion: Bry.

TURNED: See Weak.

ULCERS about, in varicose veins, hard at circumferenc
               and very sensitive: Lach.

VEINS: See Ulcers.

WALKING, A. weak, turn easily when: Carbo an., Caust.
                             Se

    Child slow in learning: Bar., *Calc.*, *Caust.*

    Cracking in joint when: Nit. ac.

    On A., feet turned (children): Brucea.

WALKING with difficulty, children: Bruc., Calc. c. an
                 p., Pinus, Sep., Sil.

    See also Pain bruised, sprained.

WEAKNESS: Aloe, Bruc., Calc., Caust., Natr., Sep.
                     Sil., Sulf.

    Turn easily while walking: Sep.

    See also Walking.

WEARINESS, unusual: Calc.

# FEET.

ACHING: Caust.

    See also Pain aching.

ACUTE: See Pain acute.

AIR, legs and, feel as if floating in (body: Apis): Sticta.

ANKLES, F. turned, children walk on: Bruc.

    See also Cold, Heaviness, Swelling.

ANT hill, F. feel as if on a: Salycil. ac.

ARTHRITIC swelling: Bufo.

    See also Pain arthritic.

ASLEEP, fall: Coccul., Col., Lyc., Sec.

        Soles: Nux.

        When sitting: Coccul., Sec.

    Feel as if dead or: *Lyc.*

    See also Moving.

BACK, boring: Mez., Nitrum.

    Burning on and in soles: Hep.

        And swelling: Thuya.

        Tearing: Puls.

    Drawing in l.: Arn.

    Swelling: Lyc., Merc., Nux, *Puls.*, Thuya.

        See also Burning.

    Tearing: Graph.

        See also Burning.

    See also Instep, Pain, etc.

BALLS, tearing in heels and: Lyc.

    See also Sweat, Ulcers.

BEATEN, soles painful as if: Puls.

    Weariness and pain as if: Lauro.

BED, feet and knees icy cold in: Carbo v.

    See also Burn, Moving.

BITING and burning: Merc.

BLACK: See Pain great.

BLISTERS: See Burnt.

BLOTCHES, small, with hard scurfs on instep: Nux.

BLUE: Kali brom.
>    See also Swelling.
BODY: See Cold.
BONES: See Lancinating, Pain in.
BOOT: See Size.
BORING in back: Mez., Nitrum.
>    See also Pain boring.
BRUISED, weakness as if: China.
>    See also Pain bruised.
BRUISES, ill effects of, to soles: Arn., Led.
BUGS: See Formication.
BURN nights, must put them out of bed or find a cool place:
>                                              Sulf.
BURNING: Bell., Cann. i., SULF.
>    And biting: Merc.
>    Pricking: Apis.
>    Tearing in back: Puls.
>    Drawing and sticking through soles: Kreos.
>    In soles: Apoc. and., *Calc.*, Hep., Kali bi., *Lyc.*, Nux,
>                         *Puls.*, SULF.
>    See also Gout, Pain burning.
BURNT, look, as far as knees, are hot, red, covered with
>    blisters here and there, attended with fever
>    and intolerable pain: Ranunc. acr.
CARRION, smell like every evening, without sweat: Sil.
CHAFED: See Ulcers.
CHILBLAINS itch: Abrot., Agar., *Puls.*
CHRONIC swelling: Led., Lyc.
CLAMMY cold to knees: Carbo v., Lauro., Sep.
COLD: Bell., *Calc.*, *Carbo v.*, *Lauro.*, *Led.*, Lyc., Pic. ac.
>                    *Sep.*, Sil., TAB.
>    And swollen: Led.
>    Clammy, to knees: Carbo v., Lauro., *Sep.*
>    Constantly, and damp as though stockings were wet:
>                                              Calc.
>    F. and hands icy: Sep.
>    Prevent sleep: Aloe.
>    Before 12 P. M.: Amm.m.
>    F. to toes, also hands, body warm: Tab.
>    Icy, to knees: Sil.
>    In bed: Carbo v.
>    One hot, the other: Chel., *Lyc.*
>    Sore from a, or getting wet: Led.

COLD; Very: Natr. m.

> With headache, A. M. and P. M., icy, damp as if up to ankles in, water: Sep.

See also Sweat.

COLDNESS of, esp. toes: *Acon.*

See also Rheumatism.

Icy, of l. sole, as if standing on oil-cloth: Morph.

COOL: See Burn.

CRACK: See Drawing.

CRAMP: Caust., Colch., Pet., Sec., Sil.

In F. and legs occasionally: Sec.

Metatarsus: Euphorb.

Heels: Mag. c.

Soles: *Agar.*, Apoc. and., Bar. c., *Calc.*, *Carbo* v. *Sil.*, Zing.

> At night: Agar.

> L.: Calc.

> On walking or dancing: Bar. c.

Painful in both: Colch.

CRAMPLIKE: See Pain cramplike.

CRAMPY pain: Cina, Colch., Digitalin, Gels.

CRAWLING and fuzzy feeling in hands and: Hyperic.

See also Formication, Throbbing, Tearing.

DAMP: See Cold very, constantly.

DANCING, cramp in soles on walking or: Bar. c.

DEAD or asleep, feel as if: Lyc.

DEATH, gangrenous: Sec.

DRAGGED: Ars., Calc.

DRAWING: Arn., Bry., Caul., Kreos., Nux, *Sulf.*

Burning and sticking through soles: Kreos.

Extending to hips, with cracking in joints on every motion: Sulf.

In back of l., esp. outer half: Arn.

Sprained: Phos. ac.

Up of the: Aeth.

See also Pain drawing.

DRAWS F. up and suddenly extends them: Tanacet.

DRY: See Skin.

EXTENDED and toes flexed: Phyt.

FAINTING: See Gangrene.

FETID sweat: *Bar. c.*, Plumb., SIL.

See also Carrion, Sweat.

FEVER: See Burnt.

FIDGETY: *Sep.*, ZINC.

FLOATING: See Air.

FORMICATION of, and legs as from bugs crawling over
skin, prevents sleep: Zinc.

FUZZY feeling in hands and: Hyperic.

GANGRENOUS death: Carbo v., Sec.

  ·With trembling and fainting: Ranunc. acr.

GIVE out while walking: Carbo an.

GOUT, rheumatic, begins in, and travels upward (Led.),
with burning (Led. coldness) in
feet at night: Sulf.

    See also Pain gouty.

GROUND: See Spine.

HANDS and, icy cold: Sep.

      Go to sleep alternately: Coccul.

  Fuzzy feeling in F. and: Hyperic.

  Sleep prevented by cold F. and: Aloe.

                  Before 12 P. M.:
                      Amm. m.

HARD red-blue, green-yellow, painful swelling: Ars.

HEADACHE: See Cold very.

HEAT, violent, in soles: Apoc. and., *Sulf.*

HEAVINESS: Agar., Cyc., Kali c., Lyc., Natr. m., Pet.,
Phos., Rhus, Sep.

  And formication: Agar.

    Stiffness: Kali c.

    Swelling: Sep.

    ·Tension, while sitting: Rhus.

    Weariness: Phos.

  Great: Natr. m., Pet., Sulf.

    Esp. of ankles: Sulf.

  Paralytic: Cyc.

HEELS: Ache from long standing: Zingib.

  Blisters on: Lamium alb.

  Boring: See Os Calcis.

  Bruised, feel as if, under H. when walkiug: Led.

  Caries of, and hip joint, pus offensive: Calc. p.

    See also Os Calcis.

  Cramp in: Mag. c. ˊ

  Crawling and throbbing: Natr. c.

    As from a worm in l.: Lach.

  Digging: See Os Calcis.

HEELS; Gout, pains sore tearing: Colch.

    Ice: See Os Calcis.

    Nails: See Pain sharp.

    Os Calcis, disease of, boring, digging caries, feels like ice: Aranea.

    Pain and stinging: Val.

        Beating, with tension: Phos.

        Boring: PULS.

        In: Agar.

           Tendo-Achilles, with dyspnoea and palpitation: Natr. c.

        Severe: Coccul., Cyc.

        Sharp, like from running nails under the skin: Rhus.

        Sprain, as if, in sole near H.: Cyc.

        Sticking and tearing: Berb.

        Stitching, tearing, from ulceration of H., <night in bed, >rubbing: Amm. m.

        Tearing, with soreness, in gout: Colch.

           See also sticking, stitching.

    Pulsative stitches: Ranunc. bulb.

    Rheumatism, obstinate, >keeping H. higher than head: Phyt.

    Sharp: See Pain sharp.

    Soreness with tearing pain in gout: Colch.

        Stinging and pain: Val.

    See also Ulcers.

    Stitches, pulsative: Ran. bulb.

    Swelling: Merc.

    Tearing: Ars., Cina, Col., Merc., Rhus.

        In, and in balls of F.: Lyc.

        See also Pain tearing, stitching, sticking, Ulceration.

    Tendo-Achilles: See Pain in.

    Tension with beating pain: Phos.

    Throbbing and crawling in both: Natr. c.

    Ulceration: See Pain stitching.

    Ulcers on H. also sore spots and raw spots on F. from friction: Cepa.

    Worm crawling in l., sensation of a: Lach.

HIPS: See Drawing.

HOLLOWS, aching pain in: Rhus.

HOT: See Burnt, Cold, Coldness, Swelling.

ICY: See Cold, Coldness.

INCLINATION to stretch out: Puls.

INCREASE of size: Col.

INSENSIBILITY, numbness and stiffness: Ars.

INSTEP, small blotches on, with hard scurfs: Nux.

    Hot swelling of: Bry.

    Puffiness about: Ruta.

    See also Back, Swelling.

ITCHING of chilblains: Agar., Abrot., *Puls.*

JERKING tearing: Cup.

KNEES: See Burnt, Cold.

LACERATING See Pain Lacerating.

LANCINATING with pressure in metatarsal bones:
                              Sabina.

    See also Pain lancinating.

LEGS and F., cramp in occasionally: Sec.

        Feel as if floating in the air: Sticta.

        Pain great, skin turns black: Tarent. C.

        See also Numbness.

LIFTED high when walking: Bell.

    See also Oedematous.

MOTION of, constant: ZINC.

NEEDLES and pins: See Prickling.

NERVOUS moving of, excessive, in bed, for hours after
        retiring, and even when asleep: Zinc.

NUMBESS: Acon., Ars., Cann. i., Onos.

    And tingling in, and legs, with pain in lumbar-dor-
        sal region, constant sexual excitement,
        severe erections (Pic. ac.): Onos.

    In joints: Cann. i.

    Insensibility and stiffness: Ars.

    Weakness and weariness: Ars.

OEDEMA and exhaustion: Ars.

OEDEMATOUS, swollen, difficult to lift: Colch.

OFFENSIVE: See Carion, Smell Sweat.

OIL-cloth: See Coldness.

PAIN: Aching in hollows of: Rhus.

    Acute, sudden, in ball of r., causing one to drop to
        floor, afterward extending to knee: Ced.

    Arthritic: Arn.

    Beaten, as if, and weariness: Lauro.

    Beating, with tension in heels: Phos:

    Boring: Coccul., Crot. h., Bell., Puls.

PAIN: Boring, digging in soles: Bell.

    In heels: *Puls.*

  Bruised: BRY.

    In malleoli: Crot. h.

    See also Swelling.

  Burning, in soles: Puls.

    Lancinating and pulsative: Bufo.

    Tensive: Puls.

    See also Swelling.

  Cramplike, in heels: Crot. h.

    Sticking in l.: Natr. m.

  Cramplike: Calc. p.

  Crampy: Colcb.

  Digging, boring in soles: Bell.

  Drawing and tearing: Coleh.

    Paralytic: Acon.

  Fatigue, as from: Verat. a.

  Fearful, as from ulcers: Canth.

  Great, in F. and legs, skin turns black: Tarent. C.

  In back of: Hell., Sil.

   Balls of: Sil.

   Bones, cannot step heavily on them: Ruta.

   Heels: Agar.

   Lumbar region: See Numbness.

   R. tarso-tibial articulation, <walking: Chel.

   Sole: Cyc., Plumb.

    At rest: Aloe.

    Near heel as if sprained: Cyc.

    When walking: Led.

  Intensely violent, on attempting to walk, as if stepping on spikes, which run upward through the limbs: Cann. i.

  Intolerable: Led., Ran. acr.

    See also Burnt, Swelling.

  Lacerating in tendons: Ratan.

  Lancinating: See Burning.

  On walking: Ars.

    See also Ulcers.

  Paralytic drawing: Acon.

  Pressing, in dorsa of: Hell.

  Severe: Canth., Caul., Phyt.

    In heels: Coccul., Cyc.

PAIN; Sprained, as if: *Bry.*, Cham., *Cyc.*

         In soles near heels: Cyc.

     Or stitching in F.: Bry.

   Sticking: Natr. m., Puls.

       Cramplike, in l.: Natr. m.

     In soles, Mag. m.

     See also tearing, tensive.

   Stinging: Apis.

     See also Spine.

   Stitching or sprained, in F.: Bry.

   Sudden: See acute.

   Suppuration: *Bry.*

       See also Swelling hot.

   Tearing, drawing: Colch.

     Sticking, in heels: Berb.

   Tensive, burning, which changes to sticking on standing: Puls.

     In back of, when sitting: *Bry.*, Puls.

   Violent: Cann. i., Sec.

     See also intensely.

   Walking: See on.

   Wrenched, as, if: RHUS.

PAINFUL as if wrenched, in morning on rising: RHUS.

   Cramp in both: Colch.

     Soles: Arn.

   Soles, as if beaten: Puls.

     On walking: Led.

   See also Swelling.

PALMS: See Skin.

PARALYSIS, complete: Ars.

   See also Rheumatism.

PARALYZED feeling: Phos.

   Seem: Cham., Phos.

PARALYTIC heaviness: Cyc.

   See also Pain paralytic.

PINS and needles: See Prickling, Sweat cold.

PRESSURE with lancinating in metatarsal bones: Sabina.

   See also Pain pressing.

PRICKING and burning in: Apis.

PRICKLING sensation in soles, like pins and needles when walking, hinders motion: Bry.

PULSATIVE: See Pain burning.

RAW: See Ulcers.

RED: See Burnt, Swelling.

RHEUMATIC tearing in, and toes: Graph.

See also Gout.

RHEUMATISM and paralysis begin in F. and lower limbs and travel upward (Sulf.) with coldness (Sulf. heat): Led.

RIGID and stiff mornings: Led.

SCURF, hard, with small blotches on instep: Nux.

SENSATION as if too large: *Apis.*

See also Prickling.

SENSITIVE: See Soles.

SITTING, heaviness and tension while: *Rhus.*

See also Asleep, Pain tensive.

SIZE, increase in, so that boot became too small: Col.

SKIN of soles and palms dry: Hep., Merc. p. a., Sulf.

Turns black, with great pain in F. and legs: Tarent. C.

See also Formication.

SLEEP, F. and hands go to alternately: Coccul.

See also Formication.

SMELL like carrion every evening, without sweat: Sil.

SOFT swelling, very, of soles: China.

SOLE, tearing on inside of F. and on: Kali c.

See also Coldness, Pain sprained.

SOLES: Become sensitive on walking, corns inflame, new corns come on S. and toes: Ant. c.

Bruises, effects of, to: Arn., Led.

Burning of: *Apoc. and.*, Calc., *Lyc.*, SULF.

Fall asleep: Nux.

Heat, violent, in: Apoc. and., Sulf.

Hot: SULF.

Painful as if beaten: Puls.

On walking: Led.

Skin of, and palms dry: Hep., Merc. p. a., Sulf.

Sore on walking: Alum., Puls.

With swelling: Natr. c.

Swelling, very soft, of: China.

See also Cramp, Pain burning, Prickling, Soreness, Sweat, Ulcers.

SORE from a cold or getting wet: Led.

Sweat: Bar. c., Calc.

SORE; Soles, on walking: Alum., Puls.

> See also Spine, Ulcers.

SORENESS of soles with swelling: Natr. c.

> See also Spine.

SPIKES: See Pain intensely.

SPINE, sore, pains stinging, could not tell when foot touched ground: Apis.

SPOTS: See Ulcers.

SPRAINED drawing: Phos. ac.

> See also Pain sprained, Painful.

STICKING in soles: Mag. m.

> See also Pain sticking.

STIFF and rigid mornings: Led.

> Swollen, F. and toes feel: *Apis*, Ars.

SWEAT, Cold: Calc., Nit. ac., Squill.

> On soles, causes toes and balls of F. to be sore, as if walking on pins: Nit. ac.

Fetid: Bar. c., Lyc., Plumb., SIL.

Makes F. Sore: Bar. c., Calc., Lyc.

Offensive: Sil.

Profuse, fetid, soles burn: Lyc.

SWELL: Plumb. ac., Sil.

> As far as ankles: Sil.

SWELLING and burning in backs: Thuya.

> Heaviness: Sep.
>
> Tension of F. evenings: Bry.

Chronic: *Led.*, Lyc.

Great, of r.: Lyc.

Hot, of instep, with bruised pain on stretching out the foot, tension in F. on stepping and suppurating pain on touch: *Bry*.

In backs of: Lyc., Merc., Nux, *Puls.*, Thuya.

Of, about ankles, with intolerable pain in ankle on stepping: *Led.*

> Heels: Merc.
>
> Soles: Natr. c.

Red, hot, with tensive, burning pains, which change to a sticking on standing: Puls.

Very soft, of soles: China.

With soreness of soles: Natr. c.

SWOLLEN and stiff, F. and toes feel: *Apis*, Ars.

> Cold: *Led.*

Evenings: Bry.

Oedematous. difficult to lift: Colch.

TEARING and burning in backs: Puls.

         Crawling: Kali c.

         Tension on margin of r.: Zinc.

   In back of: Graph.

     Heels: Ars., Cina, Col., Merc.

       And balls: Lyc.

   On inside of F. and on sole: Kali c.

   Rheumatic, in F. and toes: Graph.

   Violent: Lach.

   See also Pain tearing.

TENDONS, lacerating pain in: Ratan.

TENSION and heaviness while sitting: *Rhus.*

        Swelling of F. evenings: Bry.

        Tearing on margin of r.: Zinc.

   See also Pain tensive, Swelling.

THROBBING and crawling in heels: Natr. c.

TINGLING: See Numbness.

TOO small: See Size.

TOUCH: See Swelling.

TREMBLING: See Gangrene.

TURNED, child walks on ankles: Bruc.

ULCERS on heel also sore and raw spots on F. from friction: Cepa.

   In soles of F. and toes, balls feel chafed and sore and pain when walking: Ars.

   Pains fearful as from: Canth.

WALKING: Children backward at learning: Calc.

   Soles sore on: Alum., Puls.

     Painful on: Led.

   See also Cramp, Pain intensely, Prickling, Sweat.

WATER: See Cold.

WEAKNESS as if bruised: *China.*

   Weariness and numbness: Ars.

      Uneasiness: Lyc.

WEARINESS and heaviness: Phos.

       Pain as if beaten: Lauro.

  See also weakness.

WET, sore from a cold or getting: Led.

   See also Cold.

WRENCHED: See Painful.

# TOES.

ABSCESS: See Nail abscess.

ACHING, dull, burning, in second joint of r. big: Cim.

ANKLES: See Pain agonizing.

APART, spread: Sec.

       Stretched: Lyc.

BACKS inflamed, red and swollen: Thuya.

BALLS, acute pain in, of great: Kali bi.

     Bone pain in, of great: Sep.

     Of great, painful: *Led.*, Oleand.

             Swollen, sensitiveness of soles, tendons stiff: LED.

     Violent tearing in, of l. little: Mez.

BED: See Cramp.

BENT backward or spread apart: Sec.

BONES: See Balls, Jerking.

BURNING and crawling: Berb.

     See also Aching, Corns, Itching, Sticking, Stitches.

CONSTANTLY flexed: Ars.

CORNS: Ant. c., ARN., Ran. scler., Sulf.

     As from a tight shoe: Sulf.

     Hard: ANT. C.

     Soft: SULF.

     Sore: ARN.

     With burning and soreness, esp. painful on letting foot hang down: Ran. scler.

        Bruised or aching soreness: ARN.

CRAMPLIKE drawing: Form., Plat.

CRAMPS: Calc., Carbo an., Ferr., Nux, Sep., Sulf.

     Of, and feet which come on in bed: Ferr.

     On stretching out feet: *Sulf.*

     Under: Form.

CRAWLING and burning: Berb.

DRAWING: Caul., Dig., Thuya.

     Tearing and stitches: Lyc., Nitrum.

     See also Tearing, Pain drawing.

ENVELOPED, pain in big, as if too tightly: Plat.

FEAR: See Gout.

FROZEN: See Itching.

FUZZY: See Insensible.

GOUT: ARN., Colch., Led., *Viscum.*

> Commences in r. big,: Ben. ac.

> In big, joint, pains sticking, fears to have it touched (Arn., China) or anyone come near (Arn.): Colch.

> With great fear of being approached or touched: ARN., China, *Colch.*

GOUTLIKE tearing: Graph.

GOUTY swelling: Ginseng.

> See also Pain gouty.

GRINDING: Agar.

HARD: See Nails.

HEAT: See Pain in, Redness.

HOT: See Nail abscess.

INFLAMMATION: See Nails.

INGROWING nails: Marum, Sil.

INSENSIBLE and fuzzy feeling in fingers and: Sec.

ITCHING, burning and redness of, as if frozen: Agar.

> Great of, that have been frosted: Carbo an.

LANCINATINGS: Ginseng.

LEATHER: See Sweat.

NAILS: Abscess at root of, pain as from a hot iron: Coccul.

> Become extremely thick and hard: Graph.

> Inflammation at root of, tendency to exuberant granulations: Alum., Arn., Graph.

> Ingrowing: Marum, Sil.

>> Ulcerated (r. big): Marum.

> See also Pain in.

NUMB, painful as if: Thuya.

PAIN: Acute, in balls of great: Kali bi.

> Agonizing, in wrists, fingers, ankles and: Act. spic.

> And stitches: Phos.

> Arthritic: Arn.

> Boring, in great: Sil.

> Bruised: Arn., Bry.

>> As from a sprain: Pet.

>> Or sprained: Arn.

> Cutting: Cina.

PAIN: Drawing, jerking: Cic.

        On under portion: Led.

    Gouty: Calc. p.

    Heat and throbbing: Kali bi.

    Hot iron, as from: Coccul.

      See also Abscess.

    Hurt, as if: Chel.

    In all: Lach.

      Big, as if too tightly enveloped: Plat.

      Joint, heat in r. leg and knee: Apoc and.

      External tendons: Verat. a.

      Nail of big: Graph.

    Intense, in big: Plumb.

    Iron: See hot.

    Pressive: Cup.

    Rheumatoid, confined to: Graph.

    Sprained: See bruised.

    Sticking: Colch., Thuya.

        In middle: Thuya.

        See also Gout. -

    Stitching, comes and goes slowly: Amm. m., *Stann*.

    Violent, in joint of great: Led.

    <while sitting: Dig.

PAINFUL as if numb: Thuya.

    See also Balls. Tips.

PAINFULNESS: Con.

PIERCING as of splinters: Agar.

PRICKING: Con.

REDNESS and heat: Nit. ac.

          Of big: Nit. ac.

    See also Itching.

RHEUMATIC tearing: Graph.

    See also Pain rheumatoid.

SENSATION as if too large, swollen and stiff: Apis.

SENSITIVE: See Balls.

SHOE, corns as from a tight: Sulf.

SMELL: See Sweat.

SORENESS: See Corns.

SOUR: See Sweat.

SPASMODIC contractions: Rhus.

SPRAINED feeling in: Col.

    See also Pain sprained.

SPREAD apart or bent backward: Sec.

STICKING and burning in r.: Verat. a.

    Tearing in r.: Zinc.

    See also Pain sticking.

STIFF: See Ball, Swollen, Too large.

STITCH extending into: Hep.

STITCHES: Arn., Calc.

    And pain: Phos.

    Drawing and tearing: Lyc., Nitrum.

    Violent, extending into big: Hep.

    See also Pain stitching.

SWEAT between: Cob., Sil.

        Smells sour like sole leather: Cob.

SWELLING: Merc., Natr. c.

    Of, and balls of: Graph.

SWOLLEN and stiff, feel: Apis.

    See also Balls, Too large.

TEARING: Bell., China. Coccul., *Graph.,* Hep., *Kali c.,*
                *Mez.,* Nit. ac.

    Goutlike, in: *Graph.*

    In, and in first phalanx of big: *Kali c.*

    Jerking in tarsal and metatarsal bones: China.

    Violent, in balls of little: Mez.

THICK: See Nails become.

TIGHT shoe, corns as from a: Sulf.

    See also Pain in.

TIPS very painful when walking: *Kali c.*

TOO large, sensation as if T. and whole foot were, and
         stiff and swollen: Apis.

ULCERATED: See Nails.

ULCERS on T. and soles: Ars.

WALKING: See Tips.

# GENERAL SYMPTOMS.

ABDOMEN: See Weak.

ACHE: Coccul., Kreos.

Ankles, feet, fingers and toes, constantly and are stiff: Dios.

As if beaten, all limbs: Kreos.

ACHING: Acon., *Arn.*, Berb., *Calc. p.*, Cobalt., EUP. PERF., Euphr., Form., Lob. c., MERC., Myrica, *Phyt.*, RHUS, Still.

And soreness of whole body (Bapt.), bed or couch on which he lies feels too hard: ARN.

As if limbs were beaten or bruised: ARN.

Of extremities with soreness of flesh: *Eup. perf.*

Soreness, feeling of, esp. on motion: Calc. p.

See also Arthritis, Pain aching, Weak.

AIR, bad effects from dry cold: Acon

See also Asleep, Chorea.

AFFECTED parts excessively painful and sore: Hyperic.

Extremely sensitive to cold: Cist.

Hot, swollen and red: Agar.

Rigid: Bry.

AFFECTIONS, chronic, after injuries or shocks: Natr. m.

ANAEMIA, limbs cold, hands and feet swollen in: Ferr.

ARTHRITIC nodes: Bufo, Clem., Graph., Kali iod., Led., Menyanth., Still., Staph.

ARTHRITIS: Berb., Bry., Caust., Mangan. ox., Merc.

Chronic: Mangan. ox.

Drawing, darting, tearing stitches: Mangan. ox.

Esp. large joints, swelling (pale), heat, shiny redness, >warm wraps, <motion: Bry.

Large joints: Bry.

Nodosa deformans: Amm. p., Ben. ac., Calc., Guiac., Thuya.

Of weakly persons, easterly storms, limbs become distorted: Caust.

ARTHRITIS; Pale swelling of joints (Bry.), soreness and
aching and sharp pains: Merc.

Small joints: Act. spic,, Caul., Sticta.

With menstrual, hæmorrhoidal and urinal difficulties:
Berb.

ASLEEP, limbs: Graph.

Fall, and feel dead while walking in
open air: Graph.

Jerk on falling: *Bell.*, Cham., IGN.

See also Feel, Jerking, Limbs, Numb, Paralyzed,
Weak.

ASTHMA alt. with Rheumatism: Caul.

ATTACKS caused by change of weather: Hyperic.

AWAKE, involuntary motion while, cease during sleep:
Agar.

BEATEN, all limbs ache as if: Kreos.

General feeling of soreness as if: ARN., *Bapt.*,
Camph.

Limbs ache as if bruised or: Arn.

Feel: Puls.

Painful as if: Led.

See Limbs, Pain beaten, Stiffness.

BED, cannot remain in: Rhus.

See also Cold, Pain bruised, Stitches in.

BIRD'S claws: See Thrilling.

BITING: See Pain biting.

BLOOD boils: Arn.

BLUE, limbs cold and: Stram.

BLUISH, partial paralysis, legs cold and: Nux.

BODY, painful parts colder than rest of: Led.

See also Aching, Movements, Numbness, Pain and,
burning, Swelling.

BONES: Aching in, of extremities, with soreness of flesh:
*Eup. perf.*

In long, distressing: Still.

With feverish state of system and fullness and dullness of head: Form.

Affected at symphysis of sutures: Calc. p.

All, sensitive to touch, esp. of lower limbs: Mang. ac.

And joints feel bruised on motion: Agar.

Arthritic nodes: Bufo, Clem.

Bruised feeling of, and joints on motion: Agar.

See also Pain fine.

BONES; Boring in, of feet: Mez.

Frequent, painful in condyles of wrists: Carbo a.

Caries of long, suppuration thin, excoriates, >cold applications: Fluo ac.

With stabbing pains: Fluo. ac., Sil.

Crawling tearing in, of arms, extending into fingers: Cham.

Cutting, pressing, tearing deep in, running from affected joint along limbs, like an electric shock: Bell.

Drawing and jerking, slow painful, as if in, of extremities, when sitting quietly: Val.

Tearing: Mez.

In external condyles of r. femur: Col.

Of face: Kali bi.

Periosteum of, nightly: Rhod.

Paralytic, here and there as if in: Coccul.

See also Rheumatic, Sensitive.

Tearing, very violent, in middle part of long, so that they have hardly any firmness from sheer pain: Zinc.

Feel as if scraped by a knife, <nights: Phos. ac.

Fractures do not ossify: Calc. p., Symph.

Promotes union of: Calc. p., *Symphyt.*

Gnawing and sticking in long, esp. <in joints, less noticeable during motion than at rest: Dros.

See also Sensation, Shooting.

Graty nodosities: Dig.

Jerking, tearing in, of r. middle finger: Oleum an.

In metacarpal: China.

See also Drawing, Paralytic.

Lameness: See Paralyzed.

Paralytic, jerking tearing in, of upper limbs, <touch: China.

See also Sensitive.

Paralyzed lameness in almost all: Lach.

Periostitis of long, esp. tibia (l.) with burning pains <nights, soreness and swelling of periosteum: Mez.

From a bruise: Ruta.

Pressure and tearing in: Nitrum.

In, of ankles: Clem., Led.

BONES; Post-Merc. and syphilitic troubles of: Iod.

Rheumatic drawing in periosteum of long, of all limbs: Cann. s.

Sensation as if dogs were gnawing flesh from: Natr. s., *Nit. ac.*

Shooting and gnawing in shafts of: Bell.

Soreness: EUP. PERF.

In, in rheumatism of old people: *Eup. perf.*

Sticking in, of little finger: Cann. s.

See also Gnawing.

Stitches in, of hands and fingers: Phos. ac.

Severe, in, along arms, esp. forearms and metacarpals: Cham.

Tearing in, of last phalanges of fingers of r. hand. China.

In thigh: Indigo.

See also Crawling, Drawing, Jerking, Pain bone, Pressing.

BORING in knees, wrists and behind ears: Merc.

Wrists, fingers, shoulders and knees: Nitrum.

See also Pain biting.

BRAIN: See Rheumatism wandering.

BRUISE, general feeling of soreness as from a: Arn., Ruta.

Periostitis from a: Ruta.

See also Pain bruise.

BRUISED, aching as if limbs were beaten or: ARN.

And weary, limbs feel, mornings on waking: Zinc.

Feeling and heaviness of limbs: Sulf.

Weakness in limbs: Bry.

In limbs: Plumb., Sil., Val., Zinc.

Hands and feet feel, as if paralyzed: Phos. ac.

Sensation: Apis.

In limbs: Lyc., Merc., Pet.

Thighs, arms and back, as after great exertion: Oleum an.

Sore as if: Staph.

See also Bones, Drawing, Joints, Formication. Numbness.

See Pain bruised, Rheumatism, Tearing.

BURNING deep in limbs after retiring: Fagop.

Heat within and without: Bell.

In fingers and toes: Dig.

Of hands and feet: Sec.

See also Joints, Pain burning.

BURSTING feeling on letting limbs hang down: Vipera t.

BUZZING and tingling (Acon.) : Con.

CARIES: See Bones.

CATARRH alt. with rheumatism: Kali bi.

CHALKY deposits: See Gout.

CAHNGING: See Pain constantly, Tearing.

CHEST: See Rheumatism, Weak.

CHILLINESS and heaviness of arms and legs: Puls.

See also Movements, Pain burning, in, Rheumatism.

CHOREA: Arg. nit.

And hysteria, with constant movements, of limbs esp. hands: Tarent. H.

Attacks crosswise (Stram.) upper r. and lower l. or vice versa: Agar.

During sleep: Tarent. H., Zinc., Zizia.

Fidgety feet: Zinc., Zizia.

Legs: Tarent. H., Zizia.

From worms: Sil.

Hysterical, <evenings and night, constant jumping about of feet and legs as if floating in the air: Sticta.

Of r. arm and l. leg (Agar.), which are constantly in motion, cannot do anything; preceded by malaise: Tarent. H.

See also Chorea under Cord, Spine and Vertebrae.

CHRONIC affections after injuries or shocks: Natr. m.

Of Merc.: Hep., Nit. ac , Sil., Staph.

See also Gout, Rheumatism.

CIRCULATION: See Sensation.

CLAW: See Thrilling.

COALS: See Pain burning.

COLD: Extremities icy: Sep.

Feet and hands easily become: Cham.

Icy: Sec., Sep.

Gangrene of limbs: Sec.

Liability to take: Calc., Form., Sil.

Limbs blue and: Stram.

Hands and feet swollen, in anaemia: Ferr.

Oversensitive to pain (Coff., Cham.) and: Hep.

Partial paralysis, limbs bluish and: Nux.

Parts feel subjectively: Calc.

See also Affected, Knees, Wrinkled.

COLDER: See Painful.

COLDNESS: Ars.

    Icy: Sec.

    Of body and extremities: Iris.

      Limbs: Camph., Canth, Chin. ars., Dig., Phos., Stram.

    With deadness of limbs, and fingers: Sep.

    See also Numbness.

CONGESTION: See Neuralgia.

CONSCIOUS with opisthotonos: Nux.

CONSCIOUSNESS, loses, on falling: Cann. i.

CONSTANT uneasiness in all limbs: evenings: Merc.

    Weakness of all limbs: Mag. m.

    See also Chorea, Drowsiness, Pain constant.

CONSTANTLY: See pain constantly.

CONTRACTING: See Joints, Pain contracting.

CONTRACTIONS of arms and legs: Ox ac.

        Limbs: Sec.

        Muscles, esp. of l. extremities to toes: Merc. p. a.

    Spasmodic, of fingers and toes: Cup.

    Violent , of all limbs: Col.

    See also Spasmodic, Stiffness.

CONVULSIVE movements of limbs: Bell., Phos., Sec.

    See also Movements, Trembling, Twitching.

CONVULSIONS: See Pain cutting.

COORDINATION impaired: Alum., Gels.

COVERED, heat with aversion to being: Sec.

CRACKING, violent audible, on slightest motion of ankles, wrists and spine: Kali bi.

    See also Joints.

CRAMP and starting in limbs: Bufo.

    Clonic, of all limbs, like a stiffness: Ign.

    Excessively painful in limbs: Phos.

    In fingers and toes: Ferr.

      Knees, hands and feet: Plumb.

      Legs, arms and chest: Sec.

      Limbs: Hell., Opi.

    Intense, of extremities, great knots: Phyt.

    Of hands and feet: Euphorb.

    Writer's: Gels.

    See also Power, loss of.

CRAMPLIKE: See Intermittent, Jerking, Joints.

CRAMPY: See Pain crampy.

CRAWLING over extremities as from a fly, with numerous stitches: Bell.

CROSSWISE: See Chorea, Rheumatism.

CRUMBLE: See Pain fine.

CUTTING: See Pain cutting.

DARTING: See Arthritis, Pain cutting.

DEAD: See Asleep, Numb, Symptoms of, Lax.

DEADNESS: See Coldness.

DEBILITY: Arg. nit., Dig., *China.*

DECAYED: See Pain fine.

DIAGONALLY: See Symptoms.

DIARRHŒA alt. with rheumatism: Abrot.; Dulc.

> See also Pain rheumatic.

DISLOCATED, limbs feel as if, if moved rapidly: Phos.

DIFFICULTY of moving limbs: Con., Cup.

> See also Walk.

DISTORTED: See Arthritis of.

DISTORTION, spasmodic, of extremities: Cic.

> See also Jerking, Twitching.

DISTRESSING: See Bones.

DRAGGING: See Joints.

DRAWING: And tearing in fibrous tissues, joints and nerve sheaths: Rhus.

> Muscles of upper and lower extremities: Cham.

> Shifting: Puls.

In all limbs, with throbbing in small of back: Lach:

> Ankles, feet and toes: Caul.

> Feet and hands: Thuya.

Stretching in all limbs: Lyc.

Tearing and bruised sensation in all limbs: Merc.

Trembling in all limbs: Lyc.

> See also Arthritis chronic, Bone, Intermittent, Pain drawing, Rheumatism, Tearing, Violent.

DROPS: See Sensation.

DROPSY of limbs from renal troubles: Apis, Apoc. c.

DROWSINESS, constant, after shock: Nux m.

> See also Arthritis chronic, Weak.

DRY: See Skin.

EXHAUSTION alt. with activity: Aloe.

> General feeling of and languor: Bry., Gels., Pic. ac. Pimpin.

EXPRESSION, suffering: Canth.

EXTENSORS more affected than flexors: Calc. p.

FAINTLIKE sinking of strength: Caust:

FALLING with loss of consciousness: Cann. i,

FATIGUE: See Joints, Pain in, Walking.

FEVER: See Pain severe, Rheumatic.

FIDGETY: See Feet, Legs.

FINE: See Pain fine.

FLESH: See Bones aching, Joints gout.

FLY: See Crawling.

FORMICATION and numbness in limbs, feel as if bruised:

FROSTBITTEN: See Pain cold.                    [Phos.

FURY: See Pain cutting.

FUZZY feeling in limbs: *Sec.*

GAIT: See Power.

GALL: See Joints.

GANGLION (Ben. ac) on flexor tendons: Ruta.

GANGRENE, cold, of limbs: Sec.

GASTRALGIA alt. with rheumatism: Kali bi.

GASTRIC symptoms alt. with rheumatism: Abrot.

> See also Rheumatism wandering.

GLANDS: See Rheumatism gonorrhoeal.

GNAWING: See Bones gnawing, Pain fine.

GONORRHŒAL: See Rheumatism.

GOUT: Acon., Amm. p. *Ant. c.* ARN., Ars., Bry., CALC., Caust.; *Colch.,* Graph., Iod., Guiac., *Led.,* Lith. c. *Lyc.,* SIL., *Sulf.*

> Chronic: Amm. p., Ben. ac., CALC., *Lyc., Sil.,* Staph.
>> And nodosities: Amm. p., Staph.
>> With chalky deposits in Joints: *Calc.,* Lyc.
> From indigestion: Ant. c., *Lyc..,* Nux, *Puls.*
> L. big toe, pain radiates upward: Mang.
> Of habitual drinkers: Ant. c., *Nux.*
> Or rheumatism alt. with skin affections: Staph.
> Rheumatic, lithic acid deposits, waxy countenance:
>> Asparagus.
> With swelling of affected parts: Coccul.
> See also Joints, Rheumatism.

GOUTY abscess, promotes breaking of: Guiac.

> See also Pain gouty.

GRASPED: See Thrilling.

GRATY nodosities: Dig.

GRESSUS gallinaceus, knees involuntary drawn up when
walking: Ign.

GROWING pain: Guiac., Phos. ac.

HÆMORRHOIDAL: See Arthritis with.

HEAD, nodes on legs and, immense: Still.

See also Neuralgia.

HEART: See Numbness, Rheumatism alt., Trembling.

HEAT, external, but not internal: *Ign.*

With aversion to being covered: Sec.

See also Arthritis esp., Burning, Pain, Rheumatism,
articular.

HEAVINESS and bruised feeling of limbs: Sulf.

Chilliness of arms and legs: Puls.

Languor of limbs: Paeonia.

Paralytic feeling in limbs esp. upper:
Bell.

Stiffness of limbs: Acon.

Stitches in all limbs: Paris.

Weakness of all limbs: *Bry.*, Gels.

Limbs: Natr. m.

In all limbs on motion: Mez.

Of feet and hands: Bell.

Of limbs: *China.*, Graph., Hell., *Pic. ac.*, SEP.

Sensation of: Led.

Unusual, of limbs: Merc.

See also Weakness.

HEAVY, hands are as, lead: Phos. .

Limbs feel, like lead: Mag. m., Pic. ac.

See also Lead, Power.

HEREDITARY: See Rheumatism.

HOT, swollen and red, parts are: Agar.

See also Joints, Pain burning, Rheumatism, Wrink-
ICY: See Cold.                                      [led.

IMMENSE: See Nodes.

IMMOBILITY and insensibility of hands and feet: Plumb.

Paralytic: Coccul:

See also stiffness.

IMPRESSIONS, oversensitive to: Nux.

INABILITY to stand or walk: Canth., Cim.,  Dulc.

INDIGESTION, gout from: Lyc., Puls.

INFLAMMATORY: See Pain severe, Rheumatism.

INJURIES of tendons: Anac., Rhus.

See also Affections.

INSENSIBILITY of limbs: Verat. a.

    Of tips of fingers and toes: Sec.

    See also Immobility.

INTOXICATED feeling: Bufo.

INTENSE cramp of limbs, muscles drawn up into great knots: Phyt.

INTERMITTING cramplike drawing in knees, forearms, hands and fingers: Lyc.

INVOLUNTARY jerking in limbs: Merc.

    Motions of arms, and fingers and toes: Opi.

    See also Gressus, Jerking, Motion.

IRREGULAR and hurried movements of upper extremities: Agar.

IRRITATION: See Sleep.

ITCHING: See Pain biting.

JERK: See Asleep.

JERKING and distortion: Cina.

    As from an electric shock in limbs: Colch.

    Cramplike: China.

    In limbs: Natr. m., Sulf.

    Involuntary, of limbs: Merc.

    Of heart and trembling: Nux.

      Limbs: Stram.

    Single, of limbs on falling asleep: *Ign.*

    Twitching and distortion of limbs: Cina.

    See also Bones drawing, Joints jerking, Pain jerking, Tearing.

JOINTS: And bones feel bruised on motion: Agar.

    Broken, feel as if: Carbo an.

    Boring, gnawing deep in, after swelling has subsided: Aur. mur.

    Bruised feeling in: Col.

      Sore and tired out: Cham.

    Burning and swelling of all: Thuya.

      In spots about: Mangan.

    Contractions of: Plumb. ac.

    Crack: *Calc.*, Carbo an., Cham., Chel., Ginseng., Natr. m., *Pet.*

    Cracking and creaking in, painfully stiff: Coccul.

      In: Caust.

        All, on motion: Nit. ac., Plumb.

        Painful: Plumb.

    Cramplike dragging in: Paris.

JOINTS: Cutting: See Bone cutting.

    Dislocated: drawing in.

    Drawing in all, as if dislocated: Mez.

        Weary sensation in, esp. of knees, ankles and wrists: Mez.

    Extremities seem stiff and without: Pet.

    Feel as if stretched out: Mang. ox.

        Were loosely articulated: Lauro.

    Gout attacking many, in persons of vigorous constitutions; diathesis; flesh sore (Arn., Bapt., China, Eup. perf.), joints irritable, intolerance of touch (China): Colch.

    Irritable: Colch.

        See gout.

    Oedematous, swollen, cold to touch: Led.

    Painful hard nodes and concretions: Led.

        Stiffness: Coccul.

        See also Stiffness, Weakness.

    Post-mercurial and syphilitic troubles of bones and joints: Iod.

    Pressive drawing in all, esp. knees: Lyc.

    Pressure in, of elbows, fingers, knees, ankles and great toe: Natr. s.

    Sticking and tearing in shoulder and knee: Led., Natr. m.

    Smaller, affected: ACT. S., Caul., Kali bi., Led., Sticta., Dig., Zinc.

    Stiffness: Coccul., Lyc., Zinc.

        And swelling: Caust.

        Of lumbar and hip, latter feel as if beaten and painful: Staph.

        Painful: Coccul.

        With sharp lancinating pains above, always transverse not lengthwise of limb: Zinc.

    Sticking in, and tendons: *Kali c.*, Plumb.

    Stitching tearing in: Kali c.

    Stretched out, feel as if: Mang. ox.

    Swelling: Calc., Tilia.

        Hot, shiny red, of, (Bry.) complicated with pericarditis, generally<nights: Iod.

        Of, after slightest fatigue: Act. spic.

        Or no, of, or muscles: Merc.

        Rheumatic, of, with stiffness and contractions of muscles, tendons and limbs: Guiac.

JOINTS; Swollen, oedematous, cold to touch: Led.

    Puffy, like wind galls: Medorrh.

  Tearing in, esp. finger: Lyc.

  Trembling and weakness of all: Nit. ac.

  Uneasiness in: Sulf.

  Weakness and painfulness of: Aesc.

    In all: Col., Nit. ac.

  See also Arthritis, Bones, Gout, Rheumatism.

JUMPS: See Rheumatism.

KALI BI. suits men best, PULS. women.

KNEES, lies with, drawn up: Abies n.

  Swelling of hands and legs up to: Ferr.

  See also Gressus, Thrilling.

KNIFE, bones feel as if scraped by a, <nights: Phos. ac.

LAMENESS and desire to keep quiet: Bry.

  General, after sprains of ankles and wrists: Ruta.

  Of all limbs: Dros.

  Painful, as from a long walk: Verat. a.

    In arms and legs: Coccul.

  Painless: Con.

LANCINATING along inner surface of upper and lower
        limbs: Plumb.

  See also Numbness, Pain lancinating.

LANGUOR, general feeling of exhaustion and: Gels., Pic.
        ac., Pimpin.

LANGUOR: See also Heaviness, Pain rheumatic.

LASSITUDE from least exertion: Ars.

  See also Trembling.

LAX, hands tremble, limbs numb, dead and: China.

LAXITY of all limbs: China.

LEAD, limbs, esp. thighs, heavy as if, hung to them:
        China.

  See also Heavy, Power.

LEUCORRHŒA: See Pain under.

LIES: See Knees, Pain bruised.

LIMBS fall asleep: Graph., Stram.

  Feel asleep: Stram.

    Beaten: Puls.

  Hips and shoulders feel beaten: Staph.

LIVER: See Pain from, Stitches.

LIVIDITY of limbs: Ox. ac.

LOAD: See Stiffness.

MEMBRANE, mucous, paleness of: *Phos.*

MEN: See Kali bi.

MENSTRUAL: See Arthritis.

MERCURY, chronic effects of: Hep., Nit. ac., Sil.

MOTION, shuns: Caps.

MOVEMENTS, chilliness with every: *Sil.*

> Convulsive, of limbs alt. with trembling of whole Difficult: Clem.        [body: Arn.
>
> Involuntary, while awake, cease during sleep: Agar.
>
> Irregular: Agar.
>
> See also Convulsive, Involuntary.
>
> Convulsive, of groups of muscles preceed paralysis: Coccul.

MYGRATRY: See Neuralgia, Pain.

NECK: See Stiffness.

NEEDLES: See Pain cold.

NEURALGIA after operations: Cepa, Staph.

> Every night, well during day: Mag. p.
>
> Illio-scrotal: Rhod.
>
> In locomotor ataxia, pains sharp shooting as if under skin, often changing places and <motion: Agar.
>
> Malarial: Ars.
>
> Mygrating: *Apis*, Arn., Calc, caust., Caul., PULS., Sul.
>
> Of stump, fine threadlike, shooting pains: Cepa.
>
> Rheumatic, deep seated pains, wants to lie perfectly still (Bry.): Gels.
>
> > Change of weather or damp weather: Dulc., Ran. bulb.
>
> With violent congestion to head: Mellilot.
>
> See also Pain neuralgic.

NEURASTHENIA <going down stairs: Borax, Stann.

> Up stairs: Ars., Calc., Coca.

NODES on head and limbs immense: Still.

NODOSITIES: See Gout.

NUMBNESS and deadness of limbs: Bufo, China.

> Formication in limbs, feel bruised: Phos.
>
> Weakness in back and limbs: Ox. ac.
>
> Deadness and laxity of limbs, hands tremble: China.
>
> In limbs: Fagop.
>
> Of extremities, general exhaustion, vertigo, cold hands and feet, backs of hands mottled: Crot. h.

NUMBNESS of upper and lower limbs: Cup., Plumb.

> Paralytic, in limbs: Val.

> Peculiar, of whole body, with coldness and loss of motion in limbs, pains darting and lanci- nating esp. in l. lung, about heart, jerking inspiration, forced expiration by which he tries to>pain, the dyspnoea being<motion: Ox. ac.

> Trembling and lack of sensibility of limbs: Gels.

> See also Sensation.

OPISTHOTONOUS, consciousness with: Nux.

OPERATIONS, neuralgia after: Cepa, Staph.

OVARIAN: See Pain ovarian.

OVERSENSITIVE to cold: Hep., Sil.

> Impressions: Nux.

> Pain: Coff., Cham., Hep.

> And cold: Hep.

PAIN: Aching: Acon., *Bell.*, *Cobalt.*, Lob. c., MERC., *Phyt.*, RHUS.

> And sharp: Merc.: See also Arthritis.

> Stitches in muscles, but no swelling: Abrot.

> In posterior aspect of spleen: Lob. c.

> Shooting, stitching, sitting: Cobalt.

> Affects larger joints: Bry.

> Smaller joints: *Act. s.*, Kali bi., Led., Sticta.

> And stitches in muscles, but no swelling: Abrot.

> Attacks every other day: *Ars.*, CHIN. S., *Ferr.*, Lyc.

> <sweating (Merc.): *Ferr.*

> Beaten, as if or weary: Mez.

> Begins A. M.: Bry., *Nux*, Puls., Sep.

> Immediately on awaking, and becomes very intense and gradually de- creases (Stann.) until afternoon, when it vanishes: Sep.

> At 2 P. M., grows<until 9 P. M., is bad all night and grows better as daylight approaches: Syph.

> Biting, boring, gnawing, itching, tingling (Acon.): Ran. sc.

> BONE: Asa., *Aur.*, Bell., Calc., EUP. PERF., Hep., MERC., *Phyt.*, Rhod., *Sarsap.*, *Zinc.*

> Aching: Bell., EUP. PERF., MERC., *Phyt.*

> As if broken: EUP. PERF.

PAIN; BONE, Boring, in condyles of wrists: Carbo an.

Bruised, in, of heels: Caps.

All: Eup. perf., Ipec.

Of r. upper arm: Zinc.
Upper arm: Hep.

Paralytic, in long, and joints and small of back, on motion: Calc.

Burning, at night in, of hips and thighs: Eup. perf.

In middle of long, tendinous attachments or periosteum, also shooting, <nights (Ars., Mere.) and in damp weather (Dulc. Merc.): Phyt.

Lancinating, in, of arms: Bufo.

Cramplike, in r. metacarpal: Plat.

Digging, in tibia below l. knee: Cina.

Drawing, from elbow to fingers in: China.

In, muscles and joints: Kali bi.

Of arms at night, which does not permit sleep: Caust.

Of thigh, as if periosteum had been scraped with a knife: China.

Esp. in periosteum of: Mez., Rhod.

<cold weather, >motion, extremities esp. feet cold: Rhod.

Fine stinging and gnawing, in long, they feel bruised and as if they would crumble like decayed wood: Bell.

Gnawing and sticking, in long: Dros.
See also fine.

In all: Staph.

Ball of great toe: Sep.

Face, particularly in superior maxilliary: Calc. p.

Forepart of tibia, like chilliness, not >by heat: Colch.

Great trochanter, while walking: Cina.

Just below knee: Verat. a.

Metacarpal, of middle toes: Thuya.

Of hand, as if pounded: Bell.

Hip joint, as if flesh were loosened from: Zinc.

PAIN; BONE, in periosteum of limbs, with paralytic weakness: Cham.

Radial, as if dislocated, during rest and motion: Coccul.

Tarsal: Lach.

Neuralgic, which leaves, sore: Hep.

Paralytic bruised, in long, joints and small of back on motion: Calc.

Periosteal, rheumatic, in: Asa.

Pressive, in, of shoulders: Lauro.

Tibial: Agar.

Rheumatic in: Lact. ac.

And joints of extremities: Gels.

Esp. metacarpal, and fingers: Clem.

See also periosteal.

Shooting: See burning.

Spasmodic, in, of forearm, as if, were pressed: Verat.

L. arm: Psor.

Stabbing, in, in caries: Fluo. ac., Sil.

Stinging: See fine.

Tearing, in long: Ars.

Of last phalanges of fingers of r. hand: China.

Forearm and wrist: Thuya.

Thigh: Indigo.

Violent, in, of lower leg: Kali bi.

Weary: See beaten.

<dampness; after Merc. or syphilis: Phyt., Sarsap.

Boring and drawing, in toes, knees and forearms: Merc.

See also biting.

Bruise, resembling a, in limbs, during wet cold weather (Dulc.): Verat. a.

Bruised, as if and as if there were no strength in them: Staph.

In all limbs: Dros., Dulc., Graph.

Arms and legs: Carbo v., Cic., Con.

Upper and lower limbs: Kali bi.

Bruising: Acon., Arn.

PAIN; Burning: Acon., ARS., CANTH., *Caps.*, *Crot. h.*, KREOS., *Lyc.*, Phyt., Sep.

> Always, like red-hot coals: *Ars.*, *Kreos.*, *Lyc.*

> Stinging: Apis.

> Violent, with tearing in limbs at regular intervals, swelling of tongue, yellowness of body or only in spots: Crot. h.

> With chilliness: Caps.

> <after eating and before menses: Sep.

Changing: See constantly, wandering.

Cold neuralgic, as if produced by fine icy cold needles, with tingling (Acon., Sec.) as if frostbitten: Sac. lac.

Come and go slowly: *Stann.*, Sep.

> Suddenly: *Bell.*, Kali bi.

Confined to small spots: Calc.

Constant, contractive pressure in various parts, Pimpin.

Constantly recurring, tensive, momentary: Iris.

> Changing locations: *Lac. can.*, Lach., Magnol., PULS.

> See also Joints, Wandering.

Crampy, as if parts were screwed down in a vise: tends to be paroxysmal, <r. side and motion, >rest and heat: Col.

Cutting, shooting, starting, often burning at same time leading to fury or convulsions at times: Canth.

Darting, tearing, <on motion: Phyt.

Deep seated, in neuralgia (q. v.): Gels.

Deeper in winter, more superficial in summer: Colch.

Drawing in bones, muscles and joints: Kali bi.

> Limbs: Carbo v., Caul., Hep., *Puls.*, Sil., SULF.

> In evening: Sulf.

> Pressive: Led.

> Tearing, in extremities: Acon., Ars., Bry., SULF.

Flying: Acon., Calc. p.

Gnawing: See bone, biting.

Gouty and rheumatic, esp. <sweets: Ox. ac.

> In limbs: Caust.

Great, and tremor of limbs: Merc.

PAIN: Growing: Guiac., Phos. ac.

In all parts of rump, after getting wet in rain: Calc. p.

Limbs, as if exhausted by fatigue: Verat. a.

Arms, hands and legs down to feet: Kalm.

All limbs: China.

Elbows, knees and hips: Acon.

Limbs as from a bruise: Arn.

If exhausted: Verat. a.

Changing places continually: Kalm., Puls.

From touch: Ferr.

Rages most violently at night: Plumb.

When resting them on any object: Kali c.

<after meals: Indigo.

<joints, A. M. in bed forcing him to stretch: Puls.

Muscles, early part of motion, but>continued motion: Rhus r. and t.

With stitches, but no swelling: Abrot.

Toes, feet, fingers and hands: Con.

Wrists and ankles: Cann. i.

Increases and decreases rapidly: *Bell.*, Kali bi.

Slowly: *Stann.*, Plat.

Proportionately as sweat increases: Tilia.

Intense: See begins, Rheumatism in.

Intolerable: Ars., Cham.

Itching: See biting.

Jerking: See joint jerking.

JOINTS: Affects larger: Bry.

Smaller: Atc. s., Kali bi., Caul., Led., Sticta.

All, mostly on motion.

Articular, alt. with rheumatic paralysis: Nit-rum.

Beaten, as if or weary: Mez.

In all, on motion: Nux.

Boring and pressing, in all: Clem.

Bruised paralytic, in, small of back and long bones: Calc.

In all, mornings: Phos. ac.

Limbs and, on which he does not lie; A. M. in bed: Rhus.

PAIN: JOINTS, constantly recurring and momentary, in
                 all, mostly smaller, which shift rap-
                 idly about: Iris v.
             Changing places<,: Magnol.
             See also wandering.
         Dislocated, as if: Caps.
         Drawing in bones, muscles and: Kali bi.
             Severe, shift, in Rheumatism of small.
         Gouty: Caust., Ox. ac.                    [Caul.
         In all, painful sensation of chilliness in
                 parts down to ends of fingers
                 and toes: Bell.
             As if limbs were asleep: Ipec.
         Limbs<A. M. in bed, forcing one to stretch:
                                              Puls.
         Jerking, shifting, tearing<toward night small
                 joints also violent paralytic pain,
                 cannot hold anything in hands
             And pinching, in all: Kreos.      [Colch.
         Lancinating, sharp, above always trans-
                 verse, not lengthwise of limb, with
                 stiffness: Zinc.
         Many, in, of great toes and fingers: Natr. s.
         Momentary: See constantly.
         Paralytic, and bruised sensation of all: ARN.
             In all: Led.
             See also bruised.
         Pressive, in, of knees and wrists: Led.
         Rheumatic, in bones and, of extremities: Gels.
             In nearly all: Kali bi.
                 Severe, in r. arm and r. knee,<
                     motion, no>at rest: Iris.
             Wandering,<smaller: Kali bi.
             Recurring every spring: Kali bi.
                 See also constantly.
         Severe: See drawing, rheumatic.
         Shifting: See constantly, drawing, jerking,
                                          rheumatic.
         Shooting, from muscles to: Calc. p.
         Sore in various: Lact. ac.
         Sprain, as from a, or dislocation in hip,
                                        knee: Ign.
         Tearing: See jerking.
         Tensive: See constantly.
         Throbbing, in: Led.

PAIN; Laming: Acon.

Lancinating all along inner surface of limbs: Plumb.

Lightinglike-like: Cup., MAG. P., PLUMB., Thall.
<touch: Cup.

Makes patient restless, but not>motion: Caust.

Motion, from slightest: Bry.

Neuralgic: *Ars.*, *Bell.*, Gels., *Hep.*, Kali p., *Mag. p.*,
Pip. m. Merc., *Plumb.*, Sac. lac.,
Spig.

>and not even felt during pleasant excite-
ment: Kali p., Pip. m.

In arms and legs: Ars., Plumb.

Limbs, after scarlet fever: Gels.

Like lightining, must walk the floor: Mag. c.

See also Cold. [and phos.

Ovarian, walks bent with: Col.

Oversensitive to: Cham., Coff., Hep.

And cold: Hep.

Only at night, at rest in bed or only on lying down
during day, never during active
motion: Merc. bin.

Paralytic, in hands and lower limbs: Mez.

See also jerking.

Paroxysmal, so that he cries out, evenings and esp.
nights,<in muscular part of
thighs: Plumb.

See also crampy.

Pressive, in knees and wrists: Led.

Drawing: Led.

Rages most violently in limbs at night: Plumb.

Rheumatic, all over body: Kalm.

All > pressure; affects r. side mostly;
appear suddenly, with restlessness,
motion<pains: Form.

And gouty, are esp. <sweets: Ox. ac.

>copious sweats: Natr. m.

>hard firm pressure: Col.

In arms and legs, with stiffness of feet
and ankles: Natr. m.

Limbs: Calc., Euphorb., Form.,
Ox. ac., Propy., Rhus, Val.,
Verat.

Like electric jerks,< heat of bed (Ferr.,
Led., Merc.) >walking about:
Verat. a.

PAIN; Rheumatic, No>sweats: Merc.

        Recur every spring: Kali bi.

        Resembling a bruise, in limbs, <during wet, cold weather: Verat. a.

        Similateral, wander from side to side (Lac can.) excessive debility and general languor (Paeonia): Rhus r.

Severe: Ars., Caul., Kalm., *Ox. ac.*, PLUMB.

    In legs and arms: Ars.

    Lasting a short time, occuring in small spots: Ox. ac.

    Little or no fever, swelling or other signs of inflammation: Kalm.

Semilateral: See rheumatic.

Sharp in rheumatism (q. v.): Arn.

    Spasmodic, shoot down to feet: *Col.*

    See also lancinating.

Shift suddenly from internal parts to extremities: Phyt.

Shifting, rheumatic-like, in arms, shoulders and legs: Naja.

Shooting: Ars., Calc., Cepa, Canth., Cobalt., *Magnol.*, Phyt., SULF.

    From muscles to joints: Calc. p.

    In all limbs: Magnol.

    Through limbs: Ars., Calc.

    See also Aching, bone pain, cutting, sharp.

Soreness and rawness all over body externally and internally: Canth.

Spasmodic, in all limbs: Sec.

    See also sharp, violent.

Stabbing: See bone stabbing.

Sticking or stitching: BRY., KALI C., SULF.

Stitching: Acon., BRY., Cobalt., KALI C.. SULF.

Shoulder, from liver to: Vipera t.

Sprain, as from a, in shoulder, hip and knee: Ign.

Starting: Canth.

    See also cutting.

Stinging: APIS, Bell.

    See also fine, burning.

Splinterlike: Arg. nit., Hep., *Nit. ac.*

Streaking, in hands and legs: Fogopy.

Superficial: Coleh.

    See also deeper.

PAIN; Tearing: *Acon.*, *Bry.*, Colch., Iod., Phyt., Psor.,
RHUS.

    In arms; after slightest manual labor: Iod.

    Wandering, in extremities: Psor.

    With stiffness of limbs: Phyt.

    See also jerking.

  Tensive, in limbs, early A. M.: Bry., Nux.

  Threadlike: Cepa.

    See also Neuralgia of.

  Travel downward: Kalm., Merc.

    Upward: Led., Sulf.

  Tingling: Ran. scler.

    See also biting.

  Under l. ribs with yellow leucorrhoea: Ceanothus.

  Uterine, walks bent with: Amm. m.

  Vanishes on touch and appears elsewhere: Sang.

  Violent: Agar., Arn., Colch., Crot. h., PLUMB.

    In all paralyzed parts: Agar.

    Extremities, esp. muscular part of thighs:
Plumb.

    Spasmodic, in upper and lower limbs: Phos.
Plumb.

    See also burning.

  Wandering: APIS, Bry., Caul., *Colch*, Iris., Kali bi.,
LAC C., Magnol., *Phyt.*, Psor., PULS.,
Rhus r., *Sulf.*, Zinc.

    From side to side: LAC CAN., Rhus r., Zinc.

    Patient pale and puffy: Phyt.

    Rapidly: Colch., PULS.

    See also changing, shifting, tearing.

  Weary, as if in limbs, when at rest: Pimpin.

    See also beaten.

  $<$cool damp weather,$>$moist heat: Nux m.

  $<$from heat applied to parts: Sec.

  $<$from hot poultices: *Lyc.*

  $<$nights and warmth of bed, and not$>$sweat: *Merc.*

PAINFUL, all limbs are, feel as if beaten, on motion:

  As if beaten: Led.                    Lach.

  Concussion in limbs: Arn.

  Cramps in limbs, excessively: Phos.

  Hard nodes and concretions in joints: Led.

  Lameness, as from a long walk: Verat.

  Limbs: Cina, Cup.

PAINFUL; Muscles, on motion: Sil.
> Parts colder than rest of body: *Led*.
>> See also Affected, Bones drawing, Joints painful.
>>> Lameness, Pressure, Stitches, Walk.

PAINLESS lameness: Con.

PALE: See Arthritis, Membrane, Pain wandering.

PARALYZED feeling in limbs: 'Sil.
> See also Bones, Bruised hands. Joints, Pain violent.
>> Sleep, Stiffness.

PARALYSIS of extremities: Arg. nit., Chel., Cic., Plumb.,
>>>> Verat.
>> Lower: Canth., Con.
>>> And r. arm: Cann. i.
> Hands and feet: Lauro.
> Motion: Gels.
> Partial, legs cold and bluish: Nux.
> Rheumatic, numbness and tingling alt. with articu-
>> lar pains: Nitrum.
> See also Cord etc., Pain drawing, Symptoms of.

PARALYTIC drawing in limbs: Coccul.
> Immobility: Coccul.
> See also Bones, Heaviness, Joints, Numbness, Pain
>> paralytic weakness.

PARTS hot, swollen red: Agar.
> Affected colder than rest of body: Led.

PAROXYSMAL: See Pain paroxysmal.

PERSPIRATION, effects of checked: Rhus.
> See also Rheumatic, Sweat.

PERIOSTEUM: See Bone.

PILES alt. with rheumatism: Abrot.

PINCHING pressure in limbs, fingers and toes. as if bones
>> were crushed: Oleand.

PLAYING piano: See Power.

POST-MERCURIAL and syphilitic troubles of bones and
>> joints: Iod.

POWER, loss of: Gels.. Crot. h.
> And muscular control of extremities, hands
>> very tired from playing panio; writer's
>> cramp; gait staggering; lower limbs
>> feel heavy like lead: Gels.

PRESSURE in r. shoulder and elbow, and l. knee: Natr.s.
> Painful sticking, in muscles of extremities, in every
>> position: Dros:
> See also Pain constant, Pinching.

PROMOTES union of fractures: Calc. p., SYMPHYT.

PROSTRATION: Acon., Kali bi., *Phos.*

    Of all limbs: Agar., Colch., Puls.

      Muscular system: Verat.

    See also Trembling.

PUFFY, but little redness: Ferr. p.

    See also Pain wandering.

PUFFINESS, of a pale slightly pinkish color: Merc.

PULLING jerks and shocks in limbs: Bell.

RAWNESS: See Pain soreness.

RECURRING: See Pain constantly.

REDNESS: See Parts, Rheumatism, Swelling.

RESTING: See Pain in limbs.

RESTLESS: See Pain makes.

RESTLESSNESS, internal: *Sil.*

RHEUMATIC fever, pain increases as sweat increases:
                           Tilia.

    See also Pain, Paralysis, Neuralgia.

RHEUMATISM: Abrot., *Acon.*, *Act. s.*, Aeth., Agar., Anis, *Apis*, Apoc. and., *Arn.*, *Ars.*, Asparagus, Bellis, *Ben. ac.*, BRY., *Calc. c.* and *p.*, *Caul.*, CIM.. Clem., COLCH., Dulc., *Eup. perf.*, FERR., Ferr. pic., *Ferr. p.,* Form., Iod., *Kali bi.* and iod., KALM., Lac can., *Lith. c.*, *Lyc.*, Magnol., *Mag.c.*, Mangan., Merc. bin. and sol., Phos. ac., *Phyt.*, Pix liq., Pothos, PULS., Ran. bulb., Ran. scler., Rhod., RHUS RAD., RHUS TOX., *Salycil. ac.*, *Sang.*, Sil., Sticta, SULF., Thuya, Verat., Zinc.

    Acute: Abrot., Acon., *Apis*, Apoc. and., Ars., Bellis, Form., Merc., *Salycil. ac.*, *Sang.*, *China.*

    Articular, inflammatory, motion impossible:
                  Salycilic ac.

    Inflammatory: Abrot., Acon., *Apis*, *China*,
                      *Salycil. ac.*

    Muscular, on touching parts pain vanishes and appears elsewhere: Sang.

    With great stiffness: Apoc. and.

    Alt. with asthma: Caul.

        Catarrh: Kali bi.

        Diarrhœa: Abrot., Dulc.

*12

RHEUMATISM alt. with gastralgia: Abrot.

> Gastric symptoms: Kali bi.
> Heart and throat symptoms: Acon.
> Piles: Abrot.

Always>until evening and from warmth, pains<r.
> side: Lyc.

And gout, chronic, with lithic acid deposits and urinary symptoms,<fingers, wrists and big toe: Ben. ac.

> Pains esp.<sweets: Ox. ac.

Arthritic: Act. s., Asparag., Caul., Ferr. pic., Guiac., Kali bi., Led., Phyt., Puls., Salycil. ac., Sticta.

Chronic: Act. spic., Anis, Arn., Agar., BEN. AC., CALC., Caul, Dulc., GUIAC., Kali i., Led., LITH. C., Lyc., Magnol., Merc., Phos. ac., Pix liq., Pothos, Rhod., Rhus,

Hereditary: Sil.          [Tilia, Sil., SULF.

Crosswise: Mangan. ac.

> Shifting: Mangan.

Due to sudden chill, from wet cold, when body is hot:
> Bellis p.

During cold season,>warm season: Calc. p.

Esp. at beginning of cold season: Kali bi.

From getting feet wet: Puls.

> Wet all over: Rhus.

> Long continuance in water: Calc.

> Standing or working in water: Calc.

Gonorrhoeal: Cann. s., Clem., Phyt., PULS., Thuya.

> Joints swollen, red, glands swollen,<

Hereditary: Sil.          [damp weather: Phyt.

In smaller joints, pains shift and are of a severe drawing character: Caul.

Spring and summer; with cool days and cool nights
> Kali bi.

Inflammatory: Abrot., Acon., Apis, China, Salycil. ac., Stict., Verat.

> Articular, heat and circumscribed redness of joints: Sticta.

> Inability to move: Abrot.

> Of small joints with intense pain in neck and head: Sticta.

L. side mostly: Lach.

> To r.: Ben. ac., Lach.

Metastasis to heart: Iod., KALM., Spig.

RHEUMATISM mostly muscular, alt. in arms and hands, legs and feet, pains only at night at rest in bed or lying down during the day, never during active motion: Merc. bin.

Muscles feel bruised, sore, pains sharp, loss of power, local in winter, from exposure to damp and cold: Arn.

Muscular: BRY., *Cim.*, Merc. bin., *Nux*, Sang.

Of fleshy parts of muscles, <motion: BRY., Cim.

Large muscles of trunk, chest and back: Nux.

Old people: Eup. perf.

Bones sore, ankles swollen: Eup. perf.

One side only: Puls.

Small joints: ACT. S., *Caul.*, *Kali bi.*, Led., Rhod., Sticta.

Or gout alt. with skin affections: Staph.

Recurring in wet weather: Agar.

R. oftener: Lyc.

To l.: Apis, Lyc.

Shifting: Act. s., APIS, CIM., China, Colch., Iod., Kali bi., KALM., Lac can., Mang. ac., Merc., PULS., Rhus r., Sulf., Zinc.

From side to side: Lac can., Rhus r., Zinc.

Shifts from extremities to back and nape of neck: Caul., Tarent.

Joint to joint, leaves first without pain: Kali s.

One joint to another without leaving first: Ferr. p.

L. shoulder down arm and toward heart: Calc.

Suddenly: Kalm.

Travels downward: Kalm., Merc.

Upward: Led., Sulf., Ben. ac.

Wandering, gastric symptoms prominent (Ant. c.), joints swollen, >pressure and moving slowly about and cold, <evenings and warmth: Puls.

Which seem to attack meninges of brain, finally heart: Iod.

Wanders or jumps from side to side alt.: Lac can.

Where there are symphysis or sutures: Calc. p.

With easy perspiration: Bry.

<or brought on by cold damp weather: Dulc., Rhod.

RIGIDITY of extremities: Merc., *Nux*, Verat.

SCRAPED: See Bones.

SENSATION as if circulation had stopped in limbs: Lact. v.

    Of electric shocks in limbs: Agar.

      Drops falling on different parts of body: Cann. i.

      Numbness about limbs: Ox. ac.

    See also Drawing, Joints pain in, Thrilling.

SENSES more acute: Caps.

SENSIBILITY: See Numbness.

SENSITIVE to open air: Coccul.

    See also Bones.

SENSITIVENESS of nervous system: China.

SHOCK, chronic affections after injury or: Natr. m.

    See also Drowsiness, Pulling.

SHUDDERING: Acon.

SICK feeling in all limbs: Nux.

    As if a cold were coming on: Hep.

SINGLE jerks of limbs on falling asleep: IGN.

SINKING of strength, faint-like: Canst.

SKIN of palms and soles very dry: Hep., Mere. p. a.,

SLEEP, limbs go to: Stram.        [SULF.

    Easily (Spinal irritation): Nux, Petrol.

    On which he lies go to, as if paralyzed: Solan. lycop.

    See also Chorea, Movements.

SORENESS aching, feeling of, esp. on motion: Calc. p.

    From a slight blow: Fagop.

    General feeling of as from a bruise: ARN., *Ruta.*

      If beaten: ARN., *Bapt.*, Camph.

    Of muscles: Phyt.

      Tendons on bending or stretching them: Calc. p.

    See also Aching, Arthritis, Bones, Bruised, Weak and.

SPASMODIC contraction and extension of limbs: Lyc.

    See also Contraction, Distortion, Pain.

SPASMS, epileptiform: Plumb.

SPRAIN, limbs easily: Rhus.

    Of ankles and wrists, general lameness after: Ruta.

    Or strain of muscles from overlifting: Arn., *Calc.*, Nux, RHUS.

    See also Lameness.

SPRING: See Pain, Rheumatism.

STAGGERING: Gels.

    See also Power.

STAND: See Inability, Weak.

STARTING in affright: *Bell.*

STICKING in fingers and toes: Kali c.

    And stitches: BRY., KALI C.

STICKING in tendons and joints: Kali c., Plumb.

    See also Bones, Pain, Pressure.

STIFFNESS and contraction of muscles, tendons and limbs, with rheumatic swelling of joints: Guiac.

    And paralyzed feeling in all limbs during and after walking, with sensation of a heavy load on nape of neck: *Rhus.*

    Immovable, of contracted parts: Guiac.

    In fingers and toes: Nitrum.

    Of fingers, toes and instep: Plumb.

        Limbs: Oleand., *Phyt.*, RHUS, Sil., Verat., *Zinc.*

            Excessive: Oleand.

            With tearing pains: Phyt.

                Aching pains: Rhus.

    See also Ache, Heaviness, Joints, Rheumatism, Torpor.

STITCHES and heaviness in all limbs: Paris.

    In region of liver: Arn., Bry., Kali c.

            Painful when turning in bed: Arn.

    Toes, shoulders and fingers and in their joints: Jumping about: Cham.            [Nitrum.

    See also Arthritis chronic, Crawling, Pain stitching, strain, Sticking, Sprain.

STOOPING gait: SULF.

STRAINS: See Sprain.

STRENGTH, progressive failure of: Acon.

    See also Sinking.

STRETCHING: China.

SUDDEN: See Pain sudden.

SUMMER: See Rheumatism.

SUPPURATION: See Bone.

SWEAT, copious, of head and neck: Calc.

            Without >: Merc.

    Night: Carbo an., CHINA, Nit. ac.

        Offensive: Carbo an.

    See also Perspiration, Rheumatic pains.

SWELLING and heat: Cim.

> Redness: Acon., Puls., Rhus, Salycil. ac.
> Bluish: Lach.
> Circumscribed: Sticta.
> Pale: Acon., Ars., Bry., Coleb.
> Shining: Bell.

Great, of dissecting wounds: Apis.

No: Ferr.

Or no: Lyc., Phyt.

> Of muscles or joints: Merc.

Shining white: Dig.

See also Arthritis, Bone, Joint, Pain, Tearing.

SWELLING of hands and feet: *Rhus*, Stram.

> And legs as far as knees
> Ferr.

SWOLLEN, hands, feet and limbs, in anaemia: Ferr.

SYMPTOMS all<dampness and lying on l. side(Merc.: r.), esp. liver: Natr. s.

> <2 and 4 A. M., mornings, from mental effort, and when sleep is broken, >unbroken sleep: Nux.

And pain, generally>by motion, sometimes pressure:
> Phos. ac.

Appear diagonally: Agar.

Generally<4 P. M.,>8 P. M., but generally weak:
> Lyc.

> <Motion, nights, from open air (Rhus), cold and wet, lying on painful side, wine and pressure, >wrapping up warmly: Sil.
> <Washing in water (Phos., Sulf.), A. M. and P. M. and at rest: Sep.
> < Wetting hands (Feet, Puls.), sweets (Arg., *Ox. ac.*), in cold, damp or hot weather: Phos.

Of paralysis of l. hand and l. leg, hand feels dead when sewing: Crot. h.

<from any motion of arms or lying on back: Spig.

<rest,>motion: RHUS, Sulf.

<thinking of them: Ox. ac., Pip. m.

<water and on washing: Nit. ac.

See also Rheumatism.

TEARING and bruised sensation in all limbs: Natr. c.

Drawing in both thighs and l. arm: Col.

In all limbs, changing from one to another: Caust.

TEARING in fingers and toes: Natr. s.

In hands and feet, at intervals: Kali bi.

L. elbow: Iod.

Limbs at regular intervals, violent burning pains, swelling of tongue, yellowness of body or only in spots: Crot. h.

Jerking in limbs: Merc.

See also Arthritis, Drawing, Pain.

TENDONS: See Ganglion, Injuries, Stiffness, Soreness.

TESTICLES sensitive and swollen: *Clem.*

THRILLING, agreeable, through arms and hands and from knees down, with sensation as if a bird's claw grasped the knees: Cann. i.

THROAT: See Rheumatism alt.

TINGLING and whirring in limbs: Sec.

See also Buzzing, Trembling.

TIRED feeling: Gels., IGN., Phos. ac., Pic. ac.

And prostrated: *Bry.*, Gels.

See also Joints.

TORPOR and unusual stiffness of limbs: Hell.

TOTTERING of lower extremities: China.

TOUCH: See Bones.

TONGUE: See Tearing.

TREMBLING: Ars., Bell., China, Stram.

And loss of power in limbs: Caust., China.

Tingling in limbs: Acon.

Convulsive, of limbs: Acon.

In all limbs: Asa., Coccul., Con.

Limbs, scarcely able to walk: Cim.

Of extremities and jerking of heart: Nux.

Hands and feet: Agar., Apis.

With great prostration: Sulf.

Knees, while sitting and walking: Led.

Limbs: Chel., Cic., *Cim.*, Merc., *Stram.*

With lassitude: *Apis.*

See also Drawing, Movements, Numbness.

TREMOR all over: *Cim.*

Of limbs, >hands of another person: Asa.

TRUNK: See Rheumatism.

TWITCHING and jerking in arms, fingers and hands: Iod.

Convulsive: Kali brom., Stram.

UNEASINESS intolerable, evenings: Caust.

See also Constant, Joints.

UNSTEADINESS: See Weakness.

VIOLENT drawing through limbs: Bry.
> See also. Contractions, Cracking.

WAKING: See Bruised and.

WALK bent: Amm. m., Arn., Col.
> > With hands pressed on painful side, in ovarian neuralgia: Col.
> > Uterine pains: Amm. m.
> Inability to, difficulty in using limbs: Con.
> See also Inability, Trembling.

WALKING, fatigued easily when: Ferr.
> See also Asleep, Gressus, Stiffness.

WATER: See Rheumatism, Wrinkled.

WAXY countenance: See Gout.

WEAK after every exertion: Lyc.
> And drowsy, feels, with much muscular soreness, and aching, esp. lower limbs: Myrica.
> At intervals: Apis.
> Limbs profoundly, and fall asleep, from nervous exhaustion, thighs ache, chest and abdomen weak: Coccul.
> So, he cannot stand up: Merc. cyan.

WEAKNESS: And bruised feeling in limbs: Bry.
> > Heaviness of all limbs: *Bry.*, Gels., Natr. m.
> > Sensation of loss of power of all limbs: Merc., Nuphar.
> > Unsteadness of ligaments: Acon.
> > Weariness in all limbs: *Calc.*, ·Cham., *Merc.*
> Great: Zinc.
> > Of limbs, after slight exertion: Cic.
> > Lower extremities and heaviness of arms: Natr. c.
> In thighs and arms: Glon.
> > Upper and lower limbs: Cup., Merc., Opi.
> Of limbs: Caust., *Cup.*, Clem., Gels., Nux, Plumb., SIL., Tarent.
> Of muscular system: Form., Gels.
> Paralytic, in all limbs: *Caust.*, Coccul.
> Tremulous: *Arg. nit.*, Crot. h.
> See also Constant, Heaviness, Numbness.

WEATHER: See Attacks, Rheumatism.

WEARINESS and bruised sensation in limbs: Chel., Clem.

Exhaustion of limbs: Acon.

In all limbs during pregnancy: Calc. p.

Of wrists and ankles: Ars.

See also weakness.

WET: See Rheumatism.

WHIRRING: See Tingling.

WOMEN: See Kali bi.

WORMS, chorea from: Sil.

WOUNDS heal with difficulty: SIL.

See also Swelling.

WRINKLED, limbs pale, cold and, as if been too long in hot water: Sec.

WRITER'S cramp: Gels.

YELLOWNESS: See Tearing.

ZINC acts after, but not with Puls.

# ACCOMPANYING SYMPTOMS.

## MIND.

ABSENTMINDED: Agnus, Apis, *Cann. i.*
ALL senses more acute: Caps.
ANGER: Aloe, *Bry.*, Cham., Lyc., Natr. m., *Nux.*
　　　Irritable: Cham.
　　　Violent outbursts of: Hep., Staph.
ANGUISH: *Ars.*, Bell., Cann. i., Hep., Sil., Verat.
　　　And restlessness: Ars.
ANXIETY: ACON., Bell., Bry., *Calc.*, Pet., Plat., Sec.
APATHY: Opi., *Phos. ac.*
APPREHENSION: Bry., Calc., Hell., Natr. c., *Rhus.*
ARROGANT: Plat.
AS if beside himself: Cham.
AVARICIOUS: Calc., Lyc., Natr. c.
CAPRICIOUS: Ars., Ign.
CONFIDENCE, want of self: Lyc.
CONFUSION: Acon., Bell., Nux, *Sulf.*
CONSCIENTIOUSNESS, delicate: Ign.
DEATH, fear of: *Acon.*, *Ars.*, Sec.
　　　Predicts day of: Acon.
DEJECTION: Acon., Hep.
DELIRIUM: Agar., *Ars.*,*Bell.*, Caul., Pet., Rhus, Stram.
DEPRESSED: Ign., Natr. m., *Puls.*, Rhus.
DESIRE to bathe in cold water: Phyt.
DESIRES company: Bism., Stram.
　　　　　Light: Stram.
　　　　　Solitude: Cact., Cic., Cyc., Ign.
　　　　　To be quiet: BRY., Gels.
DESPAIRING: *Ars.*, Cann. i., *Rhus.*
DISTRACTION: Lyc., Natr. m.
DISTRUSTFUL: Ant. c.

DULLNESS: Agar., Natr. m., *Sulf.*

           Mental, < after breakfast: Carbol. ac.

EASILY aroused to anger: Bry., Lyc., *Nux.*

EXALTATION: Cann. i.

EXHILIRATION: Ox. ac.

EXCITED: Canth., Pet.

EXPOSURE, dread of: Mag. c.

FEAR: ACON., Arn., Ars., Colch., Sec.

    Of a crowd: Acon.

        Surprise: Coccul.

      Animals or dogs: China.

      Being approached or touched: **ARN.**, *Colch.*

        Alone: Ars.

      Darkness: *Cann. i.*, Val.

      Death: ACON., Ars., Cact., Opi., Plat., *Sec.*

      Dogs or animals: China.

      Strangers: Caust.

      Thieves: *Ign.*, Natr. m.

FITFUL: Nux. m.

FORGETFULNESS: Anac., Cann. i., Lyc.

          Of old people, with vanishing of thoughts: Lyc.

FRENZY: Agar., Canth.

FRETFUL: Ars., Psor.

        Ill humored: Cham., Nux, Rhus.

FRIGHTENED: Calc.

FURY: Agar., Bell., Canth.

GLOOMY: Agar.

HALLUCINATIONS: Stram.

HASTY speech: Hep.

HOMESICK, cries all the time: Caps.

HUMOR, variable: *Acon.*, Cham., *Ign.*

IDEAS, unsteadiness of: Acon.

IMBECILITY: Bar. c.

IMPATIENCE: Acon., Carbol. ac., Cham., Cina, Ign.
                                                      Nux.

IMPERTINENCE: Graph.

INDIFFERENCE: Agar., China, Kali bi., Phos. ac., Sep.

INJURE himself, wants to: Agar.

INTOXICATION, feeling of: Anac., Ant. c., Bufo, Gels.,
                                                     . Nux.

IRRITABLE: Amm. p., BRY., CHAM., NUX, Sulf. ac.
Angry: BRY.
Beside himself: CHAM.

LANGUAGE, absurd: Bell.
Inclination to profane: Anac.

LAUGH, tendency to: Cann. i., Nux m.

LIGHT, bright, intolerable: Nux.

MEMORY weak: Bar. c., Caust., Phos. ac.

MENTAL effort<symptoms: Nux.
Excitement: Agar.
Exhaustion: Bry.
Inability to sustain, efforts: Con., Opi., Rhus.
Labor, disinclination to: *Aloe.*

MILD quiet, tearful: PULS.

MOANING: Cham.
Continuously: Carbol. ac.

MOROSENESS: Agar., Bry., Canst.

MOVEMENTS, hurried: Acon., Agar., Sulf. ac.

NERVOUS excitement: Apoc. and., Caul., Cim.

OBSTINATE: Calc., Sil., Sulf.

OVERSENSITIVENESS: Coff., Colch., *Nux.*

PEEVISH, tearful: Caust., *Cham.*, Ferr., Nit. ac.

PETULANT: Carbol. ac.

PROUD: *Plat.*

QUARRELSOME: NUX.

RAGING delirium: Acon., *Canth.*

RESTLESSNESS: *Acon., Ars.,* RHUS.

REPEATS thing said: Zinc.

SADNESS, melancholy: Sabina.
Silent: *Phos. ac.*

SELF willed: Agar., *Calc.*

SENTIMENTAL mood: *Ant. c.*

SENSATION as if sinking through bed: Rhus.

SOLICITUDE: Ars.

SPITEFUL: Arn.

STARTLED, easily: *Borax.*

STRIKES and bites: *Stram.*

TALKATIVE: *Cann. i.,* LACH., Rhus, Stram.
Of daily affairs: Bry.

THINK, incapacity to: Gels.

THINKS another person is sick: *Pct.*

        Body is broken to pieces: *Bapt.*

        He has two wills: *Anac.*

        One is double: Bapt.

THOUGHTS vanish: Apis, Nit. ac., Plant.

        Or wander: Apis.

TIME passes too slowly: *Arg. nit.*

UNEASINESS of, and body: Agar.

WEEPING: Bell., *Cyc., Ign.*, Ferr., Lith. c., *Natr. m.*, Phos., PULS.

WHINING: *Cham.*

WILFUL: *Calc.*, Ferr.

WILL power, lack of: Gels. *Pic. ac.*

---

# VERTIGO.

AIR, feels light as if flying in: Apis, *Val.*

    In open: Agar., Ars. tersulf.

BED, when turning in: Con.

    <raising in, with nausea: Coccul.

EATING, after: Puls.

FALLS backward, <on rising: Acon., Bry.

    Forward: Led.

        Or backward: Rhus.

    To l.: Aur. m., Mez.

        If looking upward, to back if stooping: Caust.

HEAD, with crawling and shivering in: Arg. met.

HEAT, with, <turning head suddenly: Calc.

LOOKING upward, <on: Caust., LAC DEF., Kali p.

LYING, when: Con.

MORNING, in: Agar.

    Early, falls over: Bov.

NOSEBLEED, followed by: Acon., Bell.

SHOCK, on regaining consciousness from: Cann. i.

STAIRS, <ascending: Calc.

STOOPING, when: Acon., Puls.

    <staggers to r.: Acon.

SUN, in bright: Agar.

VOMITING, when: Crot. t.

WATER, attempting to cross: Brom., Ferr.

WRITING, when: Form.

# SCALP.

AIR, sensitiveness of, to, even in hot weather: Psor.
Touch and cool: Hep.
ALOPECIA, S. painful: Kreos.
BURNING in S., limbs alt. hot and cold: Verat.
CONGESTION, heat and dryness, with loss of hair:
Ust. m.
COVERING, least, is intolerable: Led.
DRAFT, sensation as if a cold, blew on: Pet.
EARS, threadlike pains about S., E., face and temples:
FACE: See Ears. [Cepa.
HAIR, can scarcely bear to touch, S. so sensitive: Ars.
Feels as if grasped roughly by the hand, S. sensitive
H. is touched: China.

Standing on end, S. sore, rheumatic, feels
as if drawn tightly over skull,
shivering sensation: Merc.
Pain as if, were pulled on top of head: Mag. c.
Sensation as if, were pulled up, with drawing, pressive
pain in occiput: Col.
S. sensitive when, is combed: Kreos.
HAT, S. painfully sensitive to pressure of, it feels like a
weight: Carbo v.
ITCHING, biting as from lice, <evenings: Oleand.
NEURALGIA, fine lines of pain <pressure: Caps.
PAINFUL, with alopecia: Kreos.
PRESSURE: See Hat, Neuralgia.
RHEUMATISM of S.: Merc., See also Hair.
SENSATION: See Draft, Hair, Water.
SENSITIVE: Ars., Carbo v., China, Hep., Kreos.
See also Hat, Hair.
SHIVERING sensation over S. with rheumatism: Merc.
STIFF and swollen, feels as if: Apis.
WATER, sensation of drops of, falling on. S: Cann. i.
Ice cold, running from head down S.
to face: Bell.
WEATHER: See Air.
WEIGHT: See Hat.

# HEAD.

AUTOMATIC motions of: Hell., Zinc.

BURNING on top of: Helon., SULF.

COLDNESS on top of: CALC., Sulf.

CONGESTION to: Ferr., Bell., Graph., Lyc.. Glon.

DRAWN to one side: Stram.

DULLNESS of: Natr. m., *Nux*.

FALLS backward: Agar.

FEELS scattered about bed: BAPT.

FULLNESS in: Glon.

GOUT affecting ears and: Ferr. pic.

HEAVINESS of: Con., *Gels*.

JERKING backward and forward of: Sep.

      Violent, of: Cic.

LEAD, occiput as heavy as, while perspiring (Gels.):
              Opi.

NECK, pain from forehead runs back to: Onos.

NODES immense on limbs and: Still.

NUMBNESS of upper portion: Plat.

PAIN as if hair were pulled on top of: Mag. c.

  Threadlike, about scalp, face, ears and temples
              Cepa.

PAINFUL to touch: Merc.

PERSPIRATION<pain in occiput (Gels.): Opi.

PRESSURE in: Asarum.

SHAKING of: *Cann. i.*

SWEAT, cold: Ben. ac.

  Forehead, cold, on: Verat.

      When sleeping: Merc.

    Warm: Crot. t.

  Offensive, oily: Merc.

  Prickling on bald scalp, after meals: Cepa.

  Sour smelling: Merc.

  When sleeping: Calc.

TEMPLES, threadlike pain about: Cepa.

THROBBING in: Bell., Glon., Mellilot.

# EYES.

BLUE rings around: Ars., Calc., CINA, Natr. m., Nux, Sec., *Verat.*

BURNING in: Rhod.

>by cold water: Acon., APIS, Pic. ac.

BRILLIANT, pupils large (*Bell.*, Calc.), face red Lachnan.

COLD feeling in: Spig.

CONGESTED: *Acon.*, ARN., Bell., Kali brom.

DIM, dull: Merc.

Swimming: *Ant. t.*

Sightedness: Agar., Bell.

DISTORTED: Bell.

DOUBLE vision: Aur. m., *Bell.*, *Gels.*, Nit. ac.

Or even triple: Bell.

DRYNESS, troublesome: Euphras., Hydrast.

FIXED vision: Bry., *Camph.*, Lyc., Zinc.

FEELING of round substances or sticks in: Dios.

GIVE out when using them: Jaborand., Natr. m.

GLISTEN: Hydroc. ac., Stram.

LIDS, burn: Col.

And swell along margins: Euphras.

Droop: *Gels.*, Spig.

Heavy and stiff: Rhus.

Oedematous: Apis, Kali c., Rhus.

Swelling of: Natr. c., Rhus.

Between brows and, esp. mornings, like little bags of water: KALI C.

PROMINENT, staring and restless: Stram.

SICKLY look about: Ant. t., CINA.

SUNKEN: Sec.

SWELLING about: Phos.

YELLOW: Chel., Crot. h., Dig., Sep.

# EARS.

BELL, noise as from: Led.

BLOOD oozes from, with deafness: Crot. h.

BURN and itch: Agar.

COLDNESS or cold feeling of: Calc. p.

CRACKLING as of burning birch bark: Eup. perf.

CRACKING in, on moving jaw: Aloe.

HEARS best in a noise: *Graph.*

HISSING in: Sil.

HUMAN voice difficult to hear: *Phos.*

HUMMING in, as from a bee: Abrot.

ITCHING and dragging pain in: Phos.

MACHINERY, roaring in, as from: Hydrast.

PAIN: See Itching, Stitches.

PIANO string, noises like clang or snap of a: Lyc.

PULSATIONS and buzzing in: Zinc. ox.

RED, very: Sulf.

RINGING and roaring in: *Pet.*

  In: CHIN. S., *Ferr.*, Plat.

  L. all the time: Gamboge.

STITCHES and pain extend from E. to E.: Hep.

  From within out: Sil.

  In l.: Kali bi.

WATER, noise before, like boiling: Dig.

    Like running: Cact.

WIND storm, noise as from a: Led.

WORM, sensation as from a, in: Rhod.

# NOSE.

BLUENESS around: CINA, Kreos.

BORING in *Arum. t.*, CINA, Zinc.

DROPPING from, in open air: Lith. c.

NOSEBLEED during morning sleep: Bov.

   Straining at stool: Coff.

  Every spring: Con.

  L. side: Puls.

  Mornings: Carbo an.

  On washing face or hands, or after eating:

  R. side: Bell., Bry.    [Amm. c.

*13

NOSTRILS, eruption on r. and l. upper lips: Aphis c.
    Sore cracked and crusty: *Ant. c.*
    Squirming in r. as from a worm: Calc.
              *Natr. m*
RED, of drunkards: Lach.
VARICOSE veins of: Carbo v.
WARTS, old, on, and eyebrows: Caust.
YELLOW: Chel.

---

# FACE.

ACNE itch violently: Caust.
  Of boys: Calc. pic.
   Girls: Calc. p.
ALTERED: Aeth., Cup.
BESOTTED look: Bapt., Gels.
BLACKNESS of lips: Ars., Rhus. Verat.
BLUISH: Cup.
BLUE lips: Cup.
BROWN: Arg. nit.
CHANGEABLE: Phos.
CHEEKS yellow: Chel.
COMPLEXION sallow: Cup., Lept., Plumb., *Sep.*
CRACKED lips: Ars., *Bry.*, Caps.
DRY lips: BRY., Zinc.
EARTHY colored and puffy: Merc.
ERUPTION, copper colored: Carbo an.
    Red, pimply: Led.
FLIES are attracted to head and: Calad.
FLUSHED: Bell., Canth.
    Dark red: Bapt., Opi.
    When lying down: Acon.
    With burning cheeks: *Ferr.*
GREY: Lauro., Mez.
ITCHING of: Fagop.
LIVID: Camph.
PALE: *China*, Ferr., Puls.
  And red alternately: Acon.
  Flushing easily: *Ferr.*
  One cheek the other red: *Cham.*
  Or greenish: Carbo v.
  When rising: Acon.

PAINS, drawing in bones of: Kali bi.
PULLING at lips: Zinc.
RED lips: Sulf.
SORENESS of bones of: Carbo v.
SWEAT on, when eating: Sulf. ac,
SWOLLEN: Apis, Bry., Caps., Hell., Kali c.
   Upper: Calc.
WRINKLED as if old: Abrot., Arg. nit., Calc., Psor.,
              Sarsap.
YELLOWISH and green (Carbo v.) Iod.

---

# MOUTH.

ACCUMULATION of water in: Carbo v., Mag. m.
BURNING from, to anus: Iris.
   In: Iris, Mez.
   Scraping, peppery sensation in palate and
           fauces: Mez.
COATED white with sensitive red patches: Tarax.
CORNERS of, sore cracked and crusty: Ant. c.
DRYNESS: Bry., Ginseng., Natr. m.
FETID odor from: Caps., Merc., Sil.
GUMS bleeding: Carbo v., Merc., Staph.
    And spongy: Merc., Staph.
  Blue margins: Plumb.
  Swollen: Merc.
HOT: Borax, Colch.
PALATE wrinkled: Borax.
RAWNESS from, to stomach: Tarax.
   In: Tarax.
SALIVA, bitter: Kali bi.
  Bloody: Ars.
    Runs out of, nights: Nux, *Rhus*.
  Fetid: Dig.
  Increased: Jabor., Merc.
  Salty, tastes: Cyc.
  Stringy or ropy: Kali bi.
SCALDING in: Apis.
SMARTING in: Tarax.
SORE: Canth.
  Aphthous: Sulf. ac.

SPITS fluids out of, or squirts it across bed: Bapt.
TASTE acid: Cact.
 Bitter: *Bry.*, China, Coccul., *Kali c.*, Merc., PULS.
  After food or drink: Puls.
  Of everything except water: Acon.
   Food: Bry.
  Offensive, frequent drinks of water: Bry.
 Blood in mouth, of: China.
  Of, after cough: Ipec.
 Copperish: Merc.
 Flat: Bolet., Kali c., Pet.
 Good of nothing but rye bread: Illisium.
 Greasy: Iris.
 Long after eating, of food: Puls.
 Lost: Natr. m., Puls.
 Putrid: Caps., Pet.
   Water, as of: Caps.
 Salty: Carbo v., Cyc.
 Slimy: Abrot., Iris, Pet.
 Sour: Ign., *Nux.*
TASTE sweet, of bread: Merc.
 Sweetish: Plumb.
   A. M.: Sulf.
   Of beer: Puls.
TEETH ache constantly during night: Oleand.
      Day: Coccinella.
 Decay at crown: SIL.
   Roots: THUYA.
 Decayed, gums swollen, breath fetid: Merc.
 Dull, seem: Mez.
 Painful: Arg. nit.
 Sensitive: Merc.
 Too long, feel: Arn., Merc., Mez.
TONGUE black and cracked: Lyc.
   Coating: China, Elaps, Opi.
   Dry: Alum.
    Cracked: Verat.
   Streak down center of: Lept.
 Bloody: Lach.
 Bluish: Dig., *Mur. ac.*
 Brown: Hyos.
 Catches when protruded: Apis, Lach.

TONGUE: Clean: Ipec., Rhus.
    Cold: Carbo v.
    Cracked: Kali bi.
        And dry parched: Ail.
        At tip: Lach.
        Red: Cham.
    Dry, black, hard like bark: Arg. nit.
        Shriveled, rattles in mouth: Mur. ac.
    Mapped: Natr. m., Tarax.
    Protruded, pale swollen: Vipera t.
    Red: Bism., Kali bi.,•Rhus, Tereb., Verat.
        Dry streak down middle: Phos.
        Parched, dry, paralyzed: Hyos.
    Rough: Anac., Rhus.
    Shining: Lach., Tereb.
    Shriveled: *Mur. ac.*, Verat.
    Smooth: Kali bi.
    Triangular red tip: RHUS.
    Vessicles on borders: Apis.
        Tip: Lach.
    White: Ant. c., Bism., Puls.
        Burns like fire: Mag. m.
        Swollen, sore, ulcerated: Dig.
        Thickly coated: Ant. c., Bism.
    Withered and cold: Verat.
    Yellow, dry feals as if scalded: Psor.
        Furred: Aur. m., Hyperic.
VESSICLES about: Natr. m.
VISCID mucus in: Natr. m., Phos. ac., Puls.

---

# THROAT.

COLD sensation in: Cepa.
CLOSED, T. and larynx feel as if: Lach.
DRYNESS of: Aesc., Ars., *Bell.*, Ginseng., Mag. c.
    Swelling and sticking pains: Acon.
DYSPHAGIA, mornings: Ox. ac.
FISH bone, sensation of a, or sliver in: *Arg. nit.*, *Hep.*,
                           Nit. a c.
GLOSSY looking: Cist.
GOITRE: Cist., Calc., Ferr., Iod., Spong.
PAINS, fiery, burning in oesaphagus: Verat. v.

PRESSURE on or in, as from a ball: Paris.
ROUGHNESS and soreness in: Phyt.
SORE, raw, scratches: Cobalt.
>When not swallowing: *Caps.*, *Ign.*, Led.
>With stiff neck: *Lachnan.*
STITCHES in, when not swallowing: Caps.
TIGHT around, can endure nothing: *Lach.*
WORM, squirming in, as from a: Hyperic.

---

# APPETITE AND THIRST.

APPETITE canine: Bar., Calc., *Cann. i.*, Iod., Lyc., Merc., Psor., Staph., *Sulf.*
>Nights: Arn.
>Capricious: *Cina.*
>Diminished or lost: Amm. p., *Arn.* (days), Ars., China, Dig., Ferr. (A. M.), Nux, Puls., RHUS, Bry.
>For nothing but bread: Gratiola.
>Good: Aloe.
>Great, after a walk: Psor.
>Voracious: Ptel.
>With weakness if not gratified: Phos.
>10 to 11 A. M.: SULF.
AVERSION to bananas: Elaps.
>Cheese: Chel.
>Drinks, hot: Ferr.
>Food: Colch., Chin. s.
>>Fat: Cyc., PULS.
>>Hot: Ferr., Merc. corr.
>Meat: Graph., Sep., Sulf.
>>Boiled: Chel.
>Milk: Sil.
>Sauerkraut: Hell.
>Sweets: Caust.
DESIRE for acids: Cistus, Phos. ac., *Verat.*
>Beans: China.
>Bitter things: Natr. m.
>Charcoal: Alum.
>Coal: Alum., Cic.
>Coffee: China.
>Drinks, cold: Phos.
>>Hot: Chel., *Lyc.*

DESIRE for earth: Alum.

   Eggs: Calc.

   Food, cold: Merc. corr., *Phos.*, Verat.

    Fat: Nux.

    Highly seasoned: Hep.

    Hot: Chel., *Lyc.*

    Liquid: Staph.

   Fruit: Verat.

   Juicy things: Phos. ac.

   Lime: Nit. ac.

   Manure: Merc. aur.

   Meat: Mag. c., Menyanth.

    Smoked: Kreos.

   Milk: Apis, Chel., Rhus, Sabad.

    Cold: Rhus.

   Oysters: Natr. m.

   Rags, clean: Alum.

   Refreshing things: Phos. ac.

   Spirits, ardent: Sel.

   Stimulants: Sulf. ac.

   Sweets: ARG. NIT., Sabad., Sulf.

THIRST: *Acon.*, Bell., *Bry.*, Colch., Nux, Rhus, *Verat.*,
                   Tilia.

   Burning: *Ars.*

   Chilliness after drinking: *Caps.*

   Evenings: Natr. m.

   Great: Kreos.

   Night, at: Ant. c.

   Quantity, large: Bism., *Bry.*, Verat.

     At long intervals: BRY.

    Small and often: *Apis*, ARS., Sabad.

   Unquenchable: Acon.

THIRSTLESS: *Apis*, Cyc., Gels., PULS., Sabad.

   With feeling of dryness in mouth; *Bry.*

# STOMACH.

COMPLAINTS from gluttony: *Ant. c.*, Cepa, Nux.
ERUCTATIONS: Carbo v., Carbol. ac.
    Cold: Con.
    Difficult, causing strangulation: Arg. nit.
    Loud: Arg. nit., Carbo v.
    Rancid: Carbo v., Graph.
    Smell like rotten eggs: Ant. t., ARN., Psor.
    Sour, early mornings: Lycop.
        Water: Niccol.
FAINTNESS at about 10 or 11 A. M.: SULF.
FEELS full of water: Kali c.
FLATULENCE of abdomen and: LYC.
FULLNESS and pressure of, after eating: Kali c.
GNAWING a.: Lith. c.
HANGS down relaxed: Ign., Sep., Staph., Tabac.
NAUSEA: *Ant. c.*, *Colch.*, IPEC., Lyc., Mag. m., *Verat.*
    Food, smell of, causes: *Colch.*
    On rising: *Bry.*
    Constant: IPEC.
    With gagging and retching: Ant. t., *Bism.*
PAINS in: *Dios.*, Lyc., Nux.
SPASMS of: Coccul., *Cup.*
VOMITING: Ant. c., ARS., *Coccul.*, IPEC., Iris, Sec.,
                    Sulf., VERAT.
    Acrid: *Iris.*
    As soon as S. is full: *Bism.*
    Bilious: *Ant. c.*
    Cold drinks>: Phos.
        From, as soon as they become warm on
              the S.: *Phos.*
    Eaten, of what has been: Ant. c., Ipec.
             Immediately: ARS.
    Fluids only: *Bism.*
    Frothy: Verat.
    Milk, sour: *Calc.*
    Mucus: Ipec.
    Solids only: *Bapt.*
    Sour: *Calc.*, IRIS, Puls.

# ABDOMEN.

BLOATED: Carbo v., Cham., Col., *Lyc.*

BRUISED soreness: *Apis.*

COLD feeling in: Colch., Grat., Pet.

COLDNESS of, and backache: Sarsap.

CRAMPS in: Cup.
               <urinating: Pallad.

CUTTING in umbilicus and lumbar vertebrae: Rheum.

DISTENDED: Abrot., TEREB.

    Hard: Calc.

FULLNESS: Kali c.

GRIPING: Cup., *Ipec.*

HEAT: Kali c., Sil.

HOT, tender and tense: Cup.

LIVER, distention in region of: Lauro.

        Pain from, to back: Yucca.

           Grinding in region of: Dios.

        Painful to touch: Bry.

PAIN colic-like about navel: Col.

        In liver and spleen: Bry.

        Violent, in umbilical region: Plumb.

RETRACTED: PLUMB.

RUMBLING: Dios., *Lyc.*

           Loud: Agar.

SENSITIVE: APIS.

SORE aching or cutting in spleen, extends to hips: Grind.

STITCHES: Kali c.

SUNKEN, flabby: Calc. p.

TENDERNESS: Bell.

TWISTING: DIOS.

VARICOSE veins on: Ham.

---

# ANUS, RECTUM AND STOOL.

ANUS, biting at: Dulc.

        Burning from mouth to: *Iris.*

           Soreness and fullness of: *Aesc.*

        Constantly open: PHOS.

        Crawling in: Croc., Ign.

        Drops falling from, sensation of: Cann. i.

ANUS; Itching of: *Aesc.*, Pet.

> Oozing from: *Phos.*, Sep.
>> Of fluid smelling like herring-brine: Calc.

> Prolapsus, during stool: *Pod.*
>> Urination: *Mur. ac.*

CONSTIPATION: Apoc. and., Lach., Lyc., NUX, SULF., *Thuya, Verat.*

> Constant desire: Aesc.

> Obstinate: Plumb.

> Stool hard like sheep's dung: Mag. m.
>> Insufficient: NUX.
>> Like little grains of coffee: Titania.

> With flatulence: Lyc.

DIARRHOEA alt. with rheumatism: Dulc.

> Cannot get done: *Merc. corr.*

> Daily: Pod.

> Like scraping of intestines: *Canth.*
>> Washings of meat: RHUS.

> Nightly: Kali c., PULS.

> Tenesmus, intolerable: *Canth.*, Caps., MERC. CORR.

RECTUM, cramp pain in: Eugenia.

> Swollen, dry, sore: AESC.

---

# URINE.

BLADDER, aching in, before and during urination: Berb.

> Catarrh of: CHIMAPH., Dulc.

> Irritable: Ben. ac., Eup. Perf.
>> From gouty diathesis: Sabina.

> Pain in, burning: *Canth.*, *Berb.*
>> Or sticking: Berb.

> Stranguary: *Canth.*, *Merc. corr.*, *Tereb.*

> Tenesmus: *Canth.*, MERC. CORR.
>> Rouses one from sleep nights: Ant. c.

> Weakness of: *Ferr. p.*, Hep.

URETHRA, burning along whole: CANN. S.

> Pains, cutting: CANTH.

> Stitches in: Cann. s.

URINATION, burning: *Canth.*, *Cann. s.*, *Berb.*

> Burning, with frequent waking and desire: Calc.

> Difficult: *Plumb.*, *Calc.*

> Frequent: Col.

URINATION; Involuntary. from habit; nightly: Equiset.
    Possible only with stool: ALUM., Mur. ac.
    Stream forked: Thuya.
        Spiral: Alum.
        Split: Rhus.
    Urging, constant: *Canth.*, Merc.
URINE brown like beer: Bry.
        Smells like horses: Ben. ac., Nit. ac.
    Dark, scanty: Nux.
        Turbid, red sediment: Lyc.
        With floating black specks: HELL.
    Decreasing: Tilia.
    Fiery, scanty: Acon.
    Orange color, deep: Absinth.
    Red, colors vessel: Pallad.
    Sand, red: Lyc.
        White: Sarsap.
    Smell like onions, scents room: Gambog.
    Smoky: *Tereb.*
    Strong, dark, acrid, scanty: Lith. c.
    Suppressed: Dig.
    With sediment of red sand in streaks: *Hyos.*

---

# CHEST.

ACHES, weak, can scarcely talk: Phos. ac.
ACHING in sternun: Pothos.
BRUISED feeling of articulations and cartilages; on
        motion coughing or breathing: Arn.
CLAVICLES, rheumatic pains in: Magnol.
CONSTRICTION of: Acon., Dig.
        On going up hill: *Ars.*, Calc.
CORD, sensation as if a, were around lower ribs, Cact:
                          Lyc.
COUGH with sticking in ribs, esp. l. side: Squill.
DIAPHRAGM: See Pain crampy.
DYSPNOEA, C. tight cannot lie down on account of: Ham.
EAR: See Stitches in.
HEAT: See Stitches in.
LYING down, oppression whenever: Oleand.

NEURALGIA begins in 1. intercostal region and extends into 1. arm, which becomes stiff, with
clenching of fingers and weight in nape of
neck: Paris.

Intercostal, <lying on well side: Nux.

OPPRESSION: Acon., Oleand; See also Lying.

PAIN: Aching: Calc. caust., Phos. ac., Pothos.

Acute, stabbing, with effusion, change of weather:
Ran. bulb.

A. M., on rising: Ran. bulb.

And tightness in: Phos.

At third costal cartilage, 1. side: Pix liq.

R. side: Anis.

Causes restless nights: Ran. bulb.

Constant, afternoon, 1. side: Ran. bulb.

Cramplike, close to shoulder, as if in C., as if everything were constricted: Plat.

Crampy, pressive, through diaphragm, when walking: Bism.

Cutting, tearing, beneath 1. nipple, extends to scap-
ular region and upper arm, <deep inspiration: Spig.

In 1. C., to 1. scapula: Sulf. ac.
Sternum, alt. with pain in hypogastrium: Aloe.

Pressing: Ran. bulb.

Pressive beneath sternum: Euphras.

Rheumatic, in clavicles: Magnol.

PLEURODYNIA: Arn., Bry., Cim., Nux, Ran. bulb.,
Sulf.

RHEUMATISM, intercostal: Ran. bulb.

Muscles sore to touch as if
pounded: ARN.

SCAPULA: See Pain, cutting in.

SHOULDER: See Pain cramplike.   Sternum pain.

SKIN sensitive and sternum painful: Ran. scler.

SORENESS in: Eup. perf.; See also Sternum.

Of walls as if sore or beaten: *Apis*, ARN.

SPASMS of C. alt. with vomiting: Cic.

STERNUM, burning like fire behind, and in lumbar
region: Lach.

Pain near, through r. mamma, extending to
back, between shoulders: Phell.

Soreness behind: Eup. perf.

See also Aching, Pain in, Skin, Stitches.

STICKING in ribs with cough, esp. l. side: Squill.

Violent, r. side: Ran. bulb.

STITCHES: Acon., Aeth., *Arn.*: Ars., Bov., BRY., KALI C., Ran. bulb., Stann., SULF.

And pressing in sternum: Ars.

Beneath r. ribs: Chel.

In l. costal region, alt. with sensation of heat coming out of l. ear: Acth.

R. ribs, alt. with same in r. groin: Bov.

Side: Arn., Bry., Kali c.

Knifelike, <l. side and bending forward: Stann.

Violent, in middle and front, on breathing: Ran. bulb.

With bruised pain: Arn.

. <motion: Acon., BRY.

TENSION in lower portion during motion and sitting, takes breath away: Agar.

TIGHT: See Dyspnoea.

WALKING: See Pain crampy.

WEAK and bruised feeling: Ran. bulb.

WEAKNESS: Arg. m., Phos. ac., Ran. bulb., Stann.

L. side: Arg. m.

---

# HEART.

APPLICATIONS, pain shifts to, from external:*Kalm.*

BAND, sensation as if squeezed by an iron: *Cact.*

BANDAGE, sensation as if squeezed by a tight: Colch.

CHOREA, cardiac, <l. side: *Cim.*

COLD water, troubles from checking rheumatism by putting extremities in: Tarent. H.

COLDNESS in region of H. with rheumatic pricking pain Kali bi.

CRAMP in: Ars.

CUTTING, shooting in region of : Calc. p.

GOUT: *Ben. ac.*

JERKING of H. and trembling of limbs: Nux.

NEURALGIA: Arg. m.

PAIN; Around: Arn., Cann. s., Fagop.

Bruised and stitches: Arn.

Cramplike, in precordial region: *Lach.*

Catching in region of: Puls.

Goes to H. from external applications: *Kalm.*

PAIN; In shocks, shooting into r. arm: *Phyt.*

    Lancinating, from H. to between shoulders: Glon.

    Pressive, in: Kali bi.

    Rheumatic, pricking, with coldness in region of H.:
        Kali bi.

    Sharp, in H., taking breath away, shoots into abdomen and stomach, pulse low: Kalm.

    Shooting, stabbing, from H. to l. scapula, causing violent breathing of H.: Kalm.

    Violent: Euphras.

PAINFUL sticking in: Cann. i.

PULSE slow: Cup. ars., *Dig.*. Kalm.

RHEUMATIC endocarditis, during rheumatic fever
        Aurum.

        Loud blowing with each heart-beat:
        Spig.

    Inflammation: Lach.

    Pericarditis: *Kalm.*, *Spig.*

        First stage: Kalm.

        With double stitches through cardiac region, long intervals between the two stitches: Anac.

RHEUMATISM: Acon., *Ben. ac.*, CIM., *Colch.*, KALM., Lach., *Lith. c.*, Rhus, Sang., SPIG.

    Acute: Acon., *Cim.*, Colch., *Kalm.*, Rhus, Sang.,
        *Spig.*

        Diseases following: Colch.

    Alt. with H. symptoms: Acon.

        Throat symptoms: Acon.

        Palpitation: Ben. ac.

    Chronic: *Ben. ac.*, Colch., Lach., LITH. C.

        Inflammation of H. from, soreness in region of H., stooping., Lith. c.

        Valvular insufficiencies from calcareous deposits: Lith. c.

    From getting wet, pain extends to l. arm (Acon., Kalm.) with valvular insufficiencies:
        Rhus.

    Late stages: Lach.

    Shifting to: Sang., Kalm.

        Esp. after external applications: Kalm.

        Painful stitches or pressing in region of:
        Sang.

    Troubles from checking, by putting extremities in cold water: Tarent. H.

SENSATION of weakness: Rhus.

SHOOTING: See Cutting.

STICKING, painful: Cann. i.

STITCHES: Anac., *Arn.*, Sang.

    And bruised pain: Arn.

        Double, with long intervals between the two: Anac.

        Painful, in region of H., during rheumatism: Sang.

TEARING in H. going into l. forearm: Amm. m.

TREMBLING of: Rhus.

WEAKNESS, sensation: Rhus.

# SLEEP AND DREAMS.

DREAMS, bad, vivid: Sil.

    Of falling from heights: Caps.

        Labor, bodily exertion, wading through snow, etc. *Rhus.*

    Robbers in the house: *Natr. m.*

    Tiresome: *Rhus.*

DROWSINESS at noon and sunset: Dros.

    Unconquerable, falls asleep whenever sitting down to rest: Nux m.

SLEEP, cannot unless legs are crossed: Rhod.

    Cold hands and feet prevent: Aloe.

    Cross on awaking: Lyc.

    Desire to, great: Apis.

    Disturbed: Bell., Cina, Merc.

    Erections, priapismatic, with: *Pic. ac.*

    Eyes half closed: Bell., Pod.

    Feels numb all over and cannot: Cim.

    Fright on awaking: Stram.

    Cross on awaking: LYC.

    Hard to awake: Arg. nit.

    Heat in head and cold feet prevent, before midnight: Amm. m.

    Moaning with: Bell., *Cham.*

    Pains>pains: *Merc.*

    Resting on hands and knees: Cina.

    Restless: Lyc., RHUS.

    Snoring: Opi.

    Wakes from often: Sulf.

    <after: Crotal h., LACH.

SLEEPINESS: Bell., Corn. c., *Nvx m.*, Opi.
>Daytime: Mag. m., Nux, *Phos.*, *Sulf.*
>Eating after: *Nux*, Phos.
>Irresistible, afternoons: *Puls.*

SLEEPLESSNESS: COFF.', *Opi.*, Sulf.
>At night: Kreos.

YAWNING and chilliness: *Natr. m.*
>Stretching: Aesc.

---

# CHILL, HEAT AND SWEAT.

CHILL alternating with heat: *Ars.*
>Begins in back, with great and severe pains: *Caps.*
>\>uncovering; thirst only during C.: IGN.
>Dry teasing cough during: *Rhus.*
>Mixed with heat: *Ars.*, Dig., *Merc.*, Nux.
>Of l. side: *Puls.*
>Patient desires to be held during: *Gels.*
>Shuddering: Kali c.
>With hunger and sense of general emptiness: Ail.

CHILLINESS and shivering after every drink: *Caps.*
>Thirst: IGN.
>Even near stove, intermingled with flushes of heat.
>>Colch.
>When exercising: Sil.
>>Leaving stove: Aloe.
>>Moving, during heat: *Nux.*
>With internal heat and perspiration: Merc.
>>Sweat: Col.

COLDNESS in gluteal region: Agar., *Calc.*
>Of feet and heat of head: *Sulf.*

HEAT and restlessness: *Acon.*
>Ascends as if cold water were poured over one: Sep.
>Aversion to, or being covered: *Sec.*
>Can only get warm in bed: Kali i.
>Dry: Acon., *Bell.*, Dulc., Sulf.
>>With sweat on waking: Samb.
>External, with chill: Dig.
>Hot steam comes out on raising bed clothes: *Bell.*
>Internal: *Ars.*, Canth.
>With aversion to uncover: *Nux.*

SWEAT, absence of: *Alum.*, *Graph.*
>And chilliness: Col.
>$>$eating: Anac.
>Breaks out suddenly and disappears again: Colch.
>Brings$>$: Apis., Nux., NATR. M.
>Cold: *Camph.*, *Sec.*
>During exertion: Merc., Psor.
>Exhausting, stains yellow: *Carbo an.*
>Inclined to: *Calc.*, *Merc.*
>Leaves patient weak, but$>$: Ars.
>Nights: CHINA, Merc., Psor.
>Offensive: Babt., Merc., *Sil.*
>On covered parts: Acon.
>>Hands when walking in open air: Agnus.
>>Sleeping or shutting eyes: Con.
>Only on uncovered parts: Thuya.
>Sour: Bry., Merc., *Nux*, Ruta, Sil.
>Sticky: *Merc.*
>With chilliness and internal heat: Merc.

# SKIN.

AFFECTED parts red, shining or tense and pale: Bry.
BLUE: Cup., Nux.
COLD: Ars., Camph., Cup., Verat.
COOL: Col.
DIRTY, greasy looking, with yellow blotches: Psor.
DRY: Alum., Graph.
FOLDS remain when, is pinched: Verat.
NETTLE rash over: Dulc.
SALLOW: Chel., Dig., Merc., Sep.
SHRIVELED: Sarsap., Sec.
WRINKLED: Sulf.

THE END.

# REGIONAL INDEX.

# ERRATA.

Outside cover, "And," binder's mistake.

Page 13, lines 42 and 43, read same as lines 6 and 7, on page 20.

Page 64, line 26, read Mouth for Must.

"　68, line 17, remedy is Tarent. H.

"　75, line 31, read ARN. for ARV.

"　83, line 4, remedy is Verat. a.

"　94, line 13, read "backward (Bell.) $<$ cold: RHUS."

"　104, line 11, read Natr. c. for Nayt. c.

"　171, line 32, remedy is Phos.

"　196, line 7, read "frequent drinks of water$>$: Bry.

"　207, line 35, "Pain$>$sleep."

Lightning Source UK Ltd.
Milton Keynes UK
UKHW011355230219
337801UK00007BA/160/P